CAMBRIDGE LIBRARY COLLECTION

Books of enduring scholarly value

History of Medicine

It is sobering to realise that as recently as the year in which On the Origin
of Species was published, learned opinion was that diseases such as typhus
and cholera were spread by a 'miasma', and suggestions that doctors should
wash their hands before examining patients were greeted with mockery
by the profession. The Cambridge Library Collection reissues milestone
publications in the history of Western medicine as well as studies of
other medical traditions. Its coverage ranges from Galen on anatomical
procedures to Florence Nightingale's common-sense advice to nurses, and
includes early research into genetics and mental health, colonial reports on
tropical diseases, documents on public health and military medicine, and
publications on spa culture and medicinal plants.

Hospital Sisters and Their Duties

Eva Charlotte Ellis Lückes (1854–1919) was a pioneer of nursing training and
friend of Florence Nightingale. In 1880, aged only twenty-six, she became
Matron of the London Hospital, the largest hospital in England, a post she
held until her death. During her time there she improved working conditions
for the nurses and trained her own staff, recognising the importance of a
knowledge of anatomy and physiology, but never losing sight of the primary
duty of a nurse to care for a patient's needs. She opposed proposals for the
registration of nurses as she believed it would endorse lower standards of
training than those she espoused. Her popular textbook for ward sisters
was first published in 1896 and provides practical advice on ward and staff
management and training of probationers, emphasising the importance of
the sister as role model and mentor to her staff. This is the 1893 third edition.

Cambridge University Press has long been a pioneer in the reissuing of out-of-print titles from its own backlist, producing digital reprints of books that are still sought after by scholars and students but could not be reprinted economically using traditional technology. The Cambridge Library Collection extends this activity to a wider range of books which are still of importance to researchers and professionals, either for the source material they contain, or as landmarks in the history of their academic discipline.

Drawing from the world-renowned collections in the Cambridge University Library and other partner libraries, and guided by the advice of experts in each subject area, Cambridge University Press is using state-of-the-art scanning machines in its own Printing House to capture the content of each book selected for inclusion. The files are processed to give a consistently clear, crisp image, and the books finished to the high quality standard for which the Press is recognised around the world. The latest print-on-demand technology ensures that the books will remain available indefinitely, and that orders for single or multiple copies can quickly be supplied.

The Cambridge Library Collection brings back to life books of enduring scholarly value (including out-of-copyright works originally issued by other publishers) across a wide range of disciplines in the humanities and social sciences and in science and technology.

Hospital Sisters and Their Duties

Eva C.E. Lückes

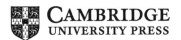

CAMBRIDGE UNIVERSITY PRESS

Cambridge, New York, Melbourne, Madrid, Cape Town,
Singapore, São Paolo, Delhi, Mexico City

Published in the United States of America by Cambridge University Press, New York

www.cambridge.org
Information on this title: www.cambridge.org/9781108053075

© in this compilation Cambridge University Press 2012

This edition first published 1893
This digitally printed version 2012

ISBN 978-1-108-05307-5 Paperback

HOSPITAL SISTERS AND THEIR DUTIES

ABERDEEN UNIVERSITY PRESS

HOSPITAL SISTERS

AND

THEIR DUTIES

BY

EVA C. E. LÜCKES

Matron to the London Hospital

AUTHOR OF "LECTURES ON GENERAL NURSING"

THIRD EDITION

LONDON

THE SCIENTIFIC PRESS, LIMITED

428 STRAND, W.C.

1893

PREFACE TO THE THIRD EDITION.

I CANNOT allow the third edition of *Hospital Sisters and their Duties* to appear, without taking this opportunity of expressing my heartfelt thanks to the many readers, both in this country and America, who have so kindly troubled themselves to write to tell me that they have found pleasure in perusing this little volume, or that such information as it contains has proved of service to them in their practical work.

While there are many admirable books on sick nursing, apparently there are none as yet which treat of those aspects of hospital life which I have attempted to deal with in the following pages. Although there must be much that can only apply in its fullest extent to the special workers for whom it is primarily intended, it is pleasant to know that the experience of others has led them in many cases to the same conclusions, and I am grateful to many, unknown to me personally, for the valuable encouragement I have received at their hands.

EVA C. E. LÜCKES.

LONDON HOSPITAL,
WHITECHAPEL, E., 19*th March*, 1893.

HOSPITAL SISTERS AND THEIR DUTIES.

CHAPTER I.

INTRODUCTORY.

IT may seem almost superfluous to add another to the many useful books on nursing already in existence, but I have not succeeded in finding one exactly adapted to meet the special want that this is intended in some measure to supply.

A trained nurse, placed in charge of wards, may seek in vain amongst the various manuals on nursing for any systematic instruction on the duties of a hospital sister, as distinct from those of a staff nurse or probationer. I hope that a few suggestions, gathered from the experience of others, may prove of service to the anxious beginner when she takes up a sister's work. Many of the inevitable difficulties may be diminished if the best method of meeting them has been carefully studied, and if the new sister is to some extent prepared for them.

People who are unacquainted with the actual, practical work of a hospital suppose, not unnaturally, that when a probationer has learnt to be a nurse she is fit to be a head nurse, or what is now gener-

1

ally termed a sister. They imagine that the satisfactory fulfilment of the duties appertaining to one position ensures the same result in the other. A better understanding of the qualifications required for a sister would immediately show that this is a very inadequate view of the subject.

I do not mean to imply that nothing has hitherto been done to help hospital sisters in the discharge of their duties. Many hints especially for them, as well as for those engaged in district or private nursing, will be found amidst the general instructions written for all nurses. But the fact remains, that much is involved in the efficient discharge of a sister's duties which appears to be but little understood. A thorough knowledge of nursing is only one out of many qualifications that are considered indispensable. It is not surprising that those who have no personal experience of hospital life should fail to perceive this, but it *is* curious that some who have had this advantage should lack sufficient penetration to discover how much is required in addition to the technical knowledge of nursing, before the satisfactory discharge of a sister's duties becomes a possibility.

Though writing for hospital sisters and nurses rather than for the general public, I wish to speak to them not of nursing, but of other duties which devolve upon them in connection with that work. All the qualities needed to make a good head of a household are essential for a good head of a ward. The same constant thought for others ; the same method in arrangement of work; the same fore-thought to meet the expected incidents of the day; the same readiness to bear the brunt of the *unexpected*, and to make the best of circumstances; the same cheerfulness and sweet temper to allay the friction so apt to rise between even good workers; the same un-failing courtesy to stray visitors of all kinds, however inopportune their visits may be,—all these and other qualities, too many and too obvious to enumerate, which go to form the guiding spirit of a well-ordered household, are at least equally indispensable in a hospital sister. The character of the sister in charge of any set of wards will not only affect the comfort and well-being of the sick or injured under her care, but will also exert a distinct influence over the members of the nursing staff who look to her for instruction and guidance.

I do not wish for one moment to exalt hospital at the expense of family life. On the contrary, I am desirous of showing the necessity for importing all the sweetest home virtues into it, and of impressing upon every woman who considers that a sister's post is the exact office to suit herself, what the nature of a sister's work really is, and what qualifications it demands from her.

If we accept the general axiom that some kinds of work are best adapted for men and some for women, we shall readily understand that women will best succeed in their own particular work by bringing into it their special characteristic of *womanliness*. I am inclined to emphasise this because

many people seem to think that if they take up
work outside their own immediate home circle, they
may dispense with the very qualities which render
them of service inside that circle, and it appears
to me that there can scarcely be a greater mistake.
We need the same qualities, and we need them rather
intensified than diminished, if they are to aid in the
achievement of really successful work. The invaluable
characteristics of which I speak will prove themselves
to be of a very strong and genuine kind if they stand
the severe test put upon them by hospital work.
They will gather strength from constant exercise,
and thus become of more value to the possessor and
of increasing service to her work. It is not difficult
to understand that if these are mere surface qualities
in the woman who comes forward to take a position
of such responsibility, her deterioration will be more
or less rapid, and her work suffer sadly, because her
character is altogether unequal to bearing the strain
put upon it.

Gentle, kindly natures may be made capable of
much good under the fostering care of watchful home
influence, even if the lovable disposition be combined
with considerable weakness; but such women are not
well fitted for hospital life. Being more dependent
upon others than upon themselves, they are overwhelmed by the constant demands made upon them,
and do not possess sufficient depth of character to
help to guide others. Such women, if thrown upon
hospital work, often make excellent subordinates,
especially if brought under the personal influence

favourable to their individual development ; but it is
not of this type of woman that the best sisters are
made. They have the right qualities, but on too
small a scale, and allied with a weakness which
renders them unadapted for responsibility. A hard,
unsympathetic person is manifestly the most unfit
of all others for work that is essentially adapted
to women who possess in a marked degree those
characteristics that we best describe as womanly.
The harder-natured women may have their special
work in other paths, no doubt, but wherever it may
be, it should never lie in a direction which brings
them in daily contact with sickness and suffering.
We cannot help others if we have no perception
of their needs, and this will be pre-eminently
the case with the woman of narrow sympathies,
who imagines that she is or could be a first-rate
sister.

Women whose sweetness and tenderness are
rooted in great strength of character, whose perception of the needs of those dependent upon them is
quick, and who are thoroughly trustworthy and
cheerfully earnest in all that they undertake—these
are the characters best fitted for the care and guidance
of others, and they will find in a hospital a splendid
opportunity for the exercise of true and noble influence towards useful ends. But I should be loath,
in an enthusiasm for nursing as woman's work, to
exalt it unduly to the disparagement of other
vocations, and particularly at the expense of the
home lives, with their round of domestic duties,

which give so much more scope than is often supposed for the development of character.

It is obvious that the kind of woman I describe
would make the best head of a household as well as
the best hospital sister, and the inadequate characters are equally insufficient in both. But as the
evil of mismanagement in a small household, while
lamentable in itself, is less deplorable than the
sight of a large family in the same condition, so in-
capacity in the person who is responsible for a large
charge is a fact to be regretted in the same proportion. A great amount of good remains undone, and
more harm is wrought by an incompetent person
undertaking public work than is ordinarily the case
if she confines her efforts to private life. It is best
that those who are incapable of giving a sufficient
response to the claims made upon them should not
accept posts which bring them in contact with large
numbers of people, but that they should exert their
influence and example for good in a more limited
circle, leaving the other appointments to be filled by
those qualified to meet the demands which will be
made upon them.

It is a mistake to suppose that there is no advantage in possessing a thorough education before entering upon hospital work, or to imagine, as some have
stated, that any general knowledge previously acquired is thrown away in a life of this kind. Familiarity with several languages, for instance, though by
no means essential, is a qualification that is certain
to prove of frequent service in the wards of any

large hospital. The cultivation of mind, which is one of the best results of a good education, is certainly not of less value to a hospital sister than to women engaged in other work. It enables her to do more for her work and to gain more from it than is otherwise possible. There are many who, in some respects, are very slow to recognise the claims which their office has upon them for the exercise of these mental and moral qualities to which I refer. The failure to perceive the many and varied directions in which their influence should be extended is naturally more marked in those who are new to the work of a sister, but, unluckily, this lack of perception is not confined to novices. In some cases many things that would be helpful to the sisters themselves and others, remain undone, not so much because these sisters lack the power to do it, as because they have failed to see the necessity or, at any rate, the desirability of exerting themselves in these directions. It is universally acknowledged that we approach a higher standard by steadily working towards an ideal, even though that ideal may be impossible of actual attainment, than we are likely to do if we are contented to take our duties mechanically, without a clear view of the possibilities that lie before us.

A sister should work with a definite determination to extend the legitimate influence which appertains to her office in every direction in which it may render good service.

I should like it to be understood that I speak with the fullest sympathy in, and regard for, all the difficulties and trials which beset the daily life and work of a hospital sister, recognising the strain which the truly noble fulfilment of her duties cannot fail to be. I am sincerely desirous of helping those who have recently entered, or who intend to enter upon this work. It will be apparent in reference to many details that I write more especially for London Hospital sisters, although I have been frequently assured that the want of a clearly defined standard of a sister's duties, as distinct from those of staff nurse or probationer, has been felt in other directions also, and doubtless many of the duties referred to are common to the post of charge nurse or hospital sister in whatever institution the appointment may be held.

Earnest workers need a definite object, upon the attainment of which they may concentrate their energies. It is encouraging to realise the great capabilities which the work of a hospital sister contains, and, at the same time, important to see in what direction lie the hindrances to its fuller development. It can scarcely be necessary to say that such criticism as is involved in the process of pointing out those errors and failings, which, in my judgment, detract from the merit and efficiency of a sister's work, is made in no unkindly spirit, and, above all, with no personal intention towards those who may be conscious that some details of their own work and management might serve as illustrations of what I regard as defects. All suggestions, to be of service, must be practical; and it would be impossible to improve any branch of hospital work from a purely theoretical point of view. Therefore we must take the subject as it exists to-day. It is only by endeavouring to understand the present condition of hospital work, and the immediate possibilities of improvement which that condition presents, that we can hope to achieve anything in the matter.

In contemplating the various branches of a sister's work, we must study in each instance what to do and what to avoid, for we can gain assistance in both directions. If only every sister would determine to resist practices that are not commendable in themselves, but which have been unreflectively followed, solely because they have been inherited from predecessors in office, that would in itself be a distinct step gained. It may be that ascertaining what is unsatisfactory in systems with which we are already familiar, is not the least important part of the task that lies before us.

With these considerations in view, it is not very remarkable that even after thorough training as a probationer, and practical familiarity with the work of a staff nurse, there is much in the duties and position of a sister that, at first, fills a novice with surprise, inasmuch as she had not previously realised to a full extent what the charge involved.

I do not mean to say that there are none, who, amidst their own work as probationers and staff nurses, possess sufficient sympathetic insight and practical observation to understand *what the sister's work means to a sister*, but those who do this will be the exceptions. For the most part they will very naturally and rightly be fully occupied with their own important duties, and be giving all their attention to what more immediately concerns themselves. Given an earnest, conscientious woman, well-grounded in nursing and showing signs of those administrative capabilities which are essential for the management of large wards, her predominant feeling in taking sister's duty for the first time is a sense of well-nigh overwhelming responsibility. She is constantly thinking: " Suppose anything goes wrong with the patients?" " Suppose the doctors are not satisfied?" " Suppose the nurses are disagreeable?" " Suppose I make mistakes in the papers for the office?" and a variety of other such-like tormenting suppositions.!

A very little experience proves that these "terrible" things are by no means certain to happen, and that if they do, the chances are very much against their happening all at once! No one entering upon such an important charge as wards containing fifty or sixty patients, as is the case with almost every individual sister at the London Hospital, could be without this sense of responsibility if she were in the least fitted to undertake it. The lack of such a feeling could but indicate that a sister had failed to perceive the nature of her appointment. Gradually this extreme sense of personal responsibility yields to custom; and it is *then*, when sisters have gained a certain amount of confidence from some proof of their own fitness which, we will hope, has come to them in the actual doing of the practical work, that their minds are free to contemplate what the office which they now fill really is, what possibilities it contains, what, in short, they mean to make of it, and how they mean to set about it and carry it on. Then, when the mechanical part of a sister's duty, if I may be allowed that expression, is nearly as familiar to her as was that of a staff nurse or probationer a few weeks previously; when the regular routine duties, which very properly absorbed most of her energies in the first instance, can be met with but little anxiety,—then is the time for each one to exert herself to study the general principles of a sister's work. She must look beyond, even whilst she fulfils the daily details with which her time is greatly occupied. She must learn to recognise the importance of what she as "sister" says and does in its immediate effect upon others, in a way that it is probable circumstances may never have rendered it necessary for her to do before.

This may seem a very simple process, and the necessity for it may appear so obvious as to render it almost superfluous to refer to it here. But I am confident that those who have been trained for two years, at any rate, and who have probably been training themselves into habits of prompt and unquestioning obedience, will admit that it requires a distinct mental effort to realise, with sufficient force for it to produce an effect upon conduct, that, whilst this obedience is still due from them to those in authority, *they* stand in a position of authority towards their subordinates that places a new and valuable influence

in their own hands. This is a fact that can never
be wisely ignored. If they do not see and use it, the
failure will shortly become evident in their inability
to exercise due control over those working under
them. Moreover, they will themselves suffer from
the loss of power involved in not using one of
the means placed at their disposal to enable the
satisfactory fulfilment of their duty as sisters. In
this direction a sense of responsibility has to be
sedulously cultivated, not checked, for the mutual
advantage of all concerned. This is the case, not
only at the beginning, when the difficulty of learning
to direct may be enhanced by a certain reluctance
on the part of the subordinates to accept the new
guidance, and when there may be need of special
tact and forbearance, but *after*, when the novelty
has worn off, when no nurse or probationer thinks
of questioning the authority of "sister," and when
it rests with her to sink to the level of average
efficiency or inefficiency, or to rise above it. A
judicious sister can render great service to the
institution to which she belongs, and extend a
beneficial influence in many directions beyond it,
through those who are sensibly and insensibly
affected by her conduct, conversation, and example
during work which brings her into personal contact
with so many.

Now, probationers are right for the most part to
devote all their energies to learning the art of nursing
itself; and if it interests them to study the system
of hospital management at the same time, as it very

reasonably may do, the fact of their inexperience may well act as a check upon their criticism. However just such criticism may be, it is still premature as coming from those who are too ignorant of the whole bearings of the case to be regarded as fair judges. I am far from having the least wish to discourage careful observation and reflection on every detail of hospital management from probationers. On the contrary, I think it most desirable that they should take an intelligent interest in the work as a whole, as well as in their individual share in it ; but it is the most thoughtful who will be the first to admit that it does not rest with them as probationers to institute reforms. They will be reasonable enough to understand that they can best forward the general work by doing with efficiency their particular part of it. They can reserve what theories they may have formed for the test of further experience and the chance of putting them into practice, if it should still seem good to them to do so, later on when opportunity offers. But sisters, without feeling themselves entitled to act in a wholly independent manner, may still be expected to look at their work from outside as well as from the standpoint of their own particular wards. They must devote their chief energies to these it is true, recognising that the welfare of the institution as a whole must depend in a great measure upon the satisfactory condition of the several parts. But, whilst giving due attention to their own portion of the work, I would have them keep very clearly before their mind what may be regarded as the general

needs for the successful working of the whole hospital.
Again, I would have them look even beyond their
own institution, and form some idea of the interests
and requirements of and from the nursing profession
in its various and ever-extending branches all over
this and other countries. Anything short of this
universal interest from sisters, at least in some degree,
is surely to be deplored. Yet some of the best sisters
will readily acknowledge, when the question presents
itself in this way, that it is a great temptation to
confine their views almost entirely to the needs of
their own wards, to the exclusion, as far as the sisters
are concerned, not only of outside interests, but even
of what may be deemed best for other parts of the
hospital. Of course, arrangements made for the good
of the whole could not be altogether dependent upon
the wishes of individual sisters. Those who will
exert themselves to look beyond their own immediate
needs, giving their cordial co-operation in the adoption
of such measures, as far as they may be in a position
to understand them, as from time to time are being
carried out, will increase their own influence by the
strength of their active helpfulness, and will have
the satisfaction of being instrumental in practically
forwarding nursing work as a whole.

From the same tendency to selfishness, if that is
not too hard a word to apply to these narrow views,
arises that species of injustice towards subordinates
which some sisters are slow to regard in this light.
I mean the sort of obstructive indifference—not to
use a harsher expression—which fails to help a new

probationer when it is not clear that any advantage
to their own particular share of the work will be
gained by it, or which would fain hinder the advancement of a promising worker to appointments outside
their own ward or hospital, because its immediate
result would be some inconvenience to the sister,
who may perhaps have helped to fit the other for
the very promotion of which she does not now
cordially approve.

We know there have been sisters—let us hope the
type may rapidly grow extinct—who would even
refrain from imparting knowledge to a probationer,
who might have the opportunity of learning from
them, just because there was no probability that they
would gain any individual credit for giving the instruction, or reap the practical benefit by having the
probationer in question long in their own particular
wards. Such a proceeding implies so low a standard
of duty that perhaps it seems scarcely worth while
to point it out as a temptation, yet it is a failing into
which many have, perhaps unconsciously, fallen in
the pressure of their daily work. Habits of this kind
are speedily formed by those who are but little inclined to look beyond themselves and their own
immediate interests, and who yet are honestly desirous of discharging their duty. I have, unfortunately,
known sisters and nurses who have been reluctant
to bestow upon others the knowledge they find useful
themselves from the smallest of all petty motives—
a desire to make their own capability contrast favour-
ably with the ignorance that is not blameworthy on

the part of a beginner, however inconvenient it may
be. It would be superfluous to make any comment
upon the narrow-minded type of character that could
refrain from teaching from such a motive, or to point
out further how unfit such women must be for sisters.
That they themselves lose much can never be doubted.
A hospital affords an excellent opportunity of proving
the truth of the old saying : " A good way of learning
is to study ; a better is to listen ; and the best is to
teach," and the most intelligent sisters have no
hesitation in pronouncing this to be the case. I am
glad to believe that such evidences of small-minded-
ness as those to which I refer are comparatively rare,
but I mention them because they are more likely
thus to be seen in their true proportions, and so
to be guarded against from the beginning. I am
inclined to the belief that those sisters who fail
most in the training of their subordinates do so
chiefly because many, with the best intentions, have
not attached sufficient importance to this duty.
They look upon it as a portion of their work to be
attended to "if there is time," or "when there is nothing else doing," and not as essentially a duty for which
time *must* be made. I am hopeful of much improvement in the general instruction given when sisters
have learnt to regard it from this point of view,
and when they begin to give the matter the large
share of their attention which its vital importance
demands.

It is only by practice that many sisters can discover the capabilities which, in all probability, they

possess for pleasantly and systematically imparting the desired knowledge. It may be that it is all simplicity itself to the sister from study and long familiarity with it; but most of it is, and will remain, a dead letter to probationers if they are left to make what use they can of experiences which, without explanation, are comparatively lost to them. For the most part, those who can teach well are not disinclined to use their powers if they realise that it is a duty. Those who cannot learn how to impart their knowledge may be capable of very good work, but should consider themselves unfitted for the post of a sister. If occupying that position, innumerable workers will necessarily suffer from their deficiencies; but these wholly incapable persons will probably be the exception. Teaching in such form as practical instruction in hospitals can best be given, *i.e.*, in the midst and during the course of the actual work that is being done, and utilising every opportunity as it offers, may seem a formidable task to those new to it; but they will find that the strangeness and the difficulty will vanish together. "I think 'Live and teach' should be a proverb as well as 'Live and learn,'" says George Eliot, and I am sure this applies to hospital sisters. "We must teach either for good or evil; and if we use our inward light, as the Quaker tells us, always taking care to feed and trim it well, our teaching must in the end be for good." There can scarcely be a nobler or more stirring incentive to make ourselves in every way worthy of a great trust than the earnest conviction that our

2

fitness is a matter of grave importance to others. The opportunity for usefulness is almost unlimited, and the extent and quality of our influence should be in proportion.

The need for efficient help is unmistakable. Physicians and surgeons are quick to feel whether their patients are being left in capable hands as far as their nursing is concerned, and whether the sister has the personal qualifications which alone can inspire confidence. Patients are almost entirely dependent upon the sister's kindly management and upon the tone that she maintains in her wards. It is not easy to define how much the patients are always seeking at her hands mentally, morally, and physically. Staff nurses and probationers are looking to her for constant guidance and learning by everything she does. It may be that all are gaining more from her example than can ever be estimated. If we remember that it is these subordinates who are the means by which the sister chiefly gets the actual nursing carried out, and that at the same time they are the links which will extend the chain of her influence in many and various directions later on, we shall gradually arrive at a juster estimate of the importance of *character* in those who aspire to be sisters.

In addition to the claims I have enumerated, the sister owes to the authorities of the institution for which she is working that conscientious discharge of duties entrusted to her which they have a right- to expect. This is a point less likely to be overlooked than many others, though in contemplating a sister's post it must not be passed over in silence. It may well be that the prospect of so full a life may not have dawned upon all who look forward to being a sister as the natural end of all hospital training, and that some help in the way of practical suggestions may be useful to those who are earnest in their desire to excel. That it takes a rare combination of qualities to fulfil all the requirements is obvious, but the more encouraging interpretation of this fact lies in the vast amount that *can* be accomplished by those who see what the demand is and lend all their energies to meet it.

To realise the need is the first step towards its fulfilment, and no slight inducement to make the steady effort involved in the attempt to meet it adequately. The power to do this can only be obtained by degrees, but then it is much to be working towards it. We may gather courage for what lies before us by remembering how others have grown up to carry with comparative freedom the full burden of their responsibilities. We may remind ourselves that the essential qualification for our own development and the attainment of a similar success is this very capacity for growth.

I have not dwelt upon the personal advantages of a sister's post as compared with that of a staff nurse or probationer because these are sufficiently evident, and I am anxious to lay all the stress possible upon what one would like to be the chief attraction in every instance—the increased means of usefulness which is ever attached to increased responsibilities.

That the added duties bring their own compensations after their kind will shortly be manifest to the sister, and that the varied results will prove a great encouragement to all earnest workers does not admit of doubt. But let us clearly understand that the efforts must be constant, whereas the results come, for the most part, in an unlooked-for direction, or at a time when we least expect them, so that we must not allow our work to be too dependent upon these results, nor enter upon it without previously counting the cost. In many respects the cost is very heavy, only it is work that in itself is so thoroughly worth doing. It is work which educates the women who are capable of being educated by it, every day of their lives. It does this by the constant exercise of all those faculties with which women are most gifted. There is urgent need for all the unselfishness, the self-sacrifice, the cheerful endurance and active sympathy which make their possessors rich in what they have to give, and their services of inestimable value to those upon whom they are bestowed. There is always much in the work of a sister to call forth these and other qualities. Would that they were always forthcoming in response to the call! If the task were not difficult, where would be the merit attached to its fulfilment of which we hear so much, and in many instances so deservedly? It may be taken as a general rule that if real credit is due to the manner in which the duties of any office are performed, infinite pains have been united to a natural capability for it. If nursing itself does not come entirely by instinct, still less will the knowledge of a sister's work, and if we are convinced that this is the case, those who aspire to excel in it will think no time wasted that is spent in fitting themselves for the task.

In dealing with this subject, I have endeavoured to put myself as far as possible in the place of a staff nurse or probationer in the London Hospital who has recently entered upon a sister's duties. I have first considered the general ward management in detail, that being a matter which claims her attention at once as one of the many new duties awaiting her. I have next dwelt at length upon the relationship which should exist between the sister and her staff nurses and probationers, to ensure the successful execution of the respective parts of their common work. I have entered into much detail concerning the methods of training probationers, because I am anxious that the subject should be better understood than it sometimes appears to be, and a juster estimate formed of its importance. It should be clearly realised that much of the efficiency with which the nursing of to-day is being carried out, and almost all the reasonable hope of the further development of it as a profession in the future, is to a great extent dependent upon the quality of the instruction now given. I am confident that if greater and more universal efforts were made by those most responsible for giving this instruction, correspondingly good results would ensue. I have devoted one chapter to the consideration of that portion of a sister's duties more immediately connected with the patients, who, it must not be forgotten, are the primary cause of her existence as a hospital worker. That the entire work of a sister admits of much greater development, that much possible good is left undone from a want of capacity or knowledge on the part of those filling the most responsible posts, is evident to all who have any practical acquaintance with the subject. When those who act as leaders to however small a number have attained a higher level and can speak from a firmer standpoint, those who are waiting below will not be slow to follow. They will climb to the same height with marvellous patience, if clear footprints have been marked out for their guidance.

The advance of everything connected with nursing, its very creation as a recognised profession for women, is of comparatively recent growth; and its present condition has not been achieved without much difficulty on the part of many of our predecessors. The rapid advance hitherto is suggestive of much that is encouraging, and it should rather inspire us to fresh effort than incline us to rest contented with what has already been gained. It seems to me that while others have had the struggle of winning the *chance* to work, when at least half their energies were expended in contending with such obstacles as prejudice and the dread of novelty strewed in their way, *we* start, as it were, with the path cleared already.

No one now seriously disputes the right of an educated woman to act as a nurse provided she shows herself competent to meet such requirements as are expected from her. The confidence of the medical profession and of the public has been gained, and there remains the splendid opportunity for women to prove themselves equal to the place which is now accorded them. It is no small privilege to have a work so suited to a woman's capacity, one that is so far removed, as it should be, from any sort of rivalry with other professions, awaiting those who are able to enter upon it. There is nothing in the nature of the work that should have any tendency to harden the sister, nothing that should narrow her sympathy, detract from her refinement, or render her less fit for the home circle. Could there be any better proof than this fact that hospital nursing is suitable work, nay, may I not say a most useful source of special and general education, for earnest, intelligent women? Those who deteriorate in it—and it must be admitted that there are such—are essentially those who did not possess the requisite qualifications for entering upon it.

I am urged to take up my present task by an intense desire to be of some service to those who have so much in their hands, and because it is possible that some help may be derived from having a few of the facts connected with the work placed distinctly before them for their consideration. I know it is very little that I can hope to accomplish, but still something may be done. To look at the work apart from ourselves, to see how we hinder it

by our selfish tendencies, either in what we do or
in what we leave undone, would help us to do our
share of work better and make us quicker to perceive
how to serve others. " He that is greatest among
you shall be your servant." If a sister could remember that this, in its degree, is what the acceptance of
her office involves, the different parts of her work
would appear in their true proportions in the light
of this illuminating thought. With Emerson, " I
see that when souls reach a certain clearness of perception, they accept a knowledge and motive above
selfishness ". To attain this perception, when it is
allied with firm determination to work earnestly, is
to ensure success.

CHAPTER II.

WHEN a sister has been duly appointed head of a ward, or rather of a set of wards, which the individual charge of each sister practically represents at the London Hospital (and it is primarily with the view of helping these sisters that I write), she cannot do better than familiarise herself with the idea that she has become, as it were, the head of a household. She is responsible within certain well-defined and unmistakable limits for the entire management of everything connected with the department which has been allotted to her, and for the arrangement, as far as her power extends, of all that contributes to the welfare of those under her charge. The habit of looking upon the wards as, to a great extent, her own, is helpful in promoting the constant interest which is needed to maintain a high standard of efficiency as a normal condition.

It is commendable for a sister to take a pride in the appearance of her wards, and though it is wise to allow each of her staff nurses a certain amount of scope for the display of their individual inclinations, she must remember that if she is the head of the household, it is only right that some evidence of her taste should prevail in the arrangements, and that she need not feel called upon to sanction what she may dislike. I mention this as some good-natured sisters occasionally speak as though the staff nurses had the supreme right to arrange details in their respective wards in accordance with their own wishes, but that does not appear a reasonable view of the matter. Sisters may be glad to gain hints from each other, and most of them will find something to admire and something of which they may disapprove in their mutual arrangements; but the desire to have their own wards as good as they can make them is perfectly legitimate, and there is no occasion for strict uniformity.

The first act on the part of a new sister should be a careful study of the standing orders that are placed in her hands on her appointment. If she is to control others and set a good example of obedience to rule, she must first ascertain carefully what her own rules are. She must make herself acquainted with the regulations which apply to staff nurses and probationers, unless she is previously familiar with them, as well as with those that have been drawn up for her own guidance. It becomes a portion of her duty as sister to enforce the due observance of all standing orders that apply to members of the nursing staff.

Everything in the wards, literally from the floor upwards, is the sister's business. I am far from meaning that she must attempt to do everything or a little of everything herself, for that would be an illustration of extremely bad management, but I wish to make it clear that the responsibility for the good condition and for the superintendence of every detail of the work rests with her. It is evident that any knowledge of housekeeping that a sister may have gained before taking up hospital work will now prove of service to her. If it unfortunately happens that she has had no experience of such matters in the past, it becomes necessary for her to remedy this defect in a woman's education with the least possible delay.

There are plenty of friends and advisers to tell a young housewife that she will never be able to manage her servants properly unless she knows something of their work. Why does it so seldom occur to people to make the same statement to the heads of wards? If a sister does not know what brass and other metals are best cleaned with; if she cannot tell whether boards have been thoroughly scrubbed with the right materials, or merely washed over; if it never occurs to her that oil-cloths must be moved for cleaning purposes, and that furniture requires to be moved before it can be swept under, how can she possibly ensure that these matters will be understood and never neglected by her subordinates? If she does not know how to clean kettles and saucepans, in what sort of a condition are they likely to be kept? If she has never troubled herself to learn what will remove different sorts of stains, how does she expect to keep her floors, tables, etc.,

free from them? If she does not know the use,
appearance, and cost of brooms, brushes, and other
domestic appliances, how can she tell whether they
have been employed for the right purpose and have
been fairly used, whether they are worn out or could
reasonably be used a little longer?

If a sister's mind is a blank on the subject of cooking, how can she see after the patients' diets with
any degree of efficiency? It is true that the actual
cooking is not done in the wards, but how can she
give a report of any value on the food that is sent up
if she is ignorant of its quality and the manner of its
preparation?

There can scarcely be a greater mistake than to
imagine that any knowledge of housekeeping and
general domestic management is thrown away in the
person who aspires to be the head of a ward. The
contrary is emphatically the case, so much so that it
becomes essential to study these things as sister, if
there has been no occasion to do it before.

She should retain as little as possible of work that
is purely mechanical in her own hands, for the purpose of bestowing her attention in such directions as
it may be required, and with the object of giving
herself time for that general superintendence of all
which is essentially the sister's work. It is not
desirable that she should spend her days in doing
work that should be done by other people, but it is
necessary that she understand exactly how everything ought to be done, otherwise she will not
always be able to enforce the *thoroughness* that is

perhaps even more important in a hospital than elsewhere.

Good results must be maintained, and perhaps a busy sister in the midst of what we familiarly term " a very heavy take-in " alone can tell with what effort from herself and some of her workers this uniformly good result is produced. It is in times of additional pressure that the good or bad management of a ward becomes most evident, and it is on such occasions that a really efficient sister will reap the reward of her method of work. However, a beginner had better lose no time in grasping the fact that whatever the unexpected difficulties are, slovenliness must not be allowed to creep in, or she will be apt to accept an excuse as sufficient explanation for a state of affairs that is in itself unsatisfactory. I am by no means wishing to imply that no excuse is adequate for anything short of the best. It is easy to conceive circumstances in which arrangements far from perfection may be the *best possible*, and therefore rather to be commended than blamed. The sister will soon learn to recognise this and refrain from unnecessary worry. But it is well that she should understand that if she is content to pass over indifferent work as good enough, and to listen too readily to the explanations of why work that should have been done well has been done badly, other people will accept a second-rate standard with surprising rapidity, and there will be increased difficulty in raising their ideas above it.

Nothing is more discouraging to first-rate workers

than contentment on the part of the sister with mediocrity. It lessens the desire to excel instead of increasing it. If the sister is a keen observer, and knows how to praise and blame with equal heartiness and discrimination, she will draw out the best work of which her subordinates are capable.

She must not expect when she has once arranged the work—say for the wardmaid—that all her trouble in that direction is at an end. On the contrary, nothing but continuous supervision will keep wardmaids and others up to the mark. It is true that if the wardmaid is a person of average capability for the class from which wardmaids are selected, she will not need to be told the same things every day, but it is very probable that what she remembers one day she may need to be reminded of the next! This is the case with most servants who have not undergone the thorough training which fits them for first-rate places, and it is scarcely reasonable to expect wardmaids to be brilliant exceptions to a general rule. At the same time, it would be unwise for a sister to expend unlimited energy and patience in a hopeless attempt to make an incompetent woman suit, or at any rate she should report her difficulty. If she has secured a wardmaid who does *what* she does well, the sister had better accept the necessity for seeing that the wardmaid's work is duly carried out, as a portion of a sister's regular duty, and not look upon what will, in most cases, prove inevitable, as an unexpected grievance.

When a sister takes up the management of a

ward, she will do well, unless previously familiar with it, to make no sudden change in any particular. It is best to let everything go on as before, while she is carefully observing all that takes place, and reflecting on what changes are needed, and on the most convenient method of *gradually* introducing them. When the sister has quite made up her mind that an improved arrangement is desirable, she should speak to those whom it may concern as pleasantly as she can, with a view of enlisting their cordial co-operation, instead of that tacit resistance with which so many unthinking people meet alterations of any kind. Any display of the obstruction which seems inherent in certain types of character is best met on the part of the sister by the patient firmness that makes it quietly evident she has no intention of yielding the point. This will ensure with the least trouble the carrying out of her wishes.

The sister is aware on taking charge that there are certain rules made for the satisfactory working of the whole institution, and that, in all respects in which these regulations are defined, it is her duty to conform to them herself, and to insist that they are duly complied with by all her subordinates. Sisters have no power to make exceptions on their own account to definite rules made for any class of workers in whatever part of the hospital they may be working, but should co-operate loyally with the authorities in seeing that these rules are invariably observed. It is well for the sister to realise in the practical arrangement of her work that her wards are part of a whole, and that while everything must be done to render that part as efficient as possible, the good of the whole must not be sacrificed to the apparent convenience of one set of wards. There is plenty of opportunity for the individuality of each sister to be displayed in those matters that are left for her to arrange in accordance with her own ideas, but it is only by the universal observance of such regulations as have been found desirable that a general condition of order and discipline can be maintained, irrespective of the efficiency or inefficiency of different sisters.

It is also helpful for the sister to know that certain lines have been laid down for the government of all. She is not left without any assistance to do the best she can with regard to the entire management of her ward, but is expected to conduct that management successfully, under conditions that leave her free to exercise her own discretion on every point where individual differences of opinion do not affect the harmonious working of the whole institution. To take an illustration of my meaning in connection with the wardmaids. They are all expected to come to their work and leave it at a fixed hour, to be given their exact time off duty, only within the limits of settled hours, to conform to certain regulations respecting the wearing of their uniform, and one or two other rules that I need not pause here to enumerate. It is manifestly desirable that these rules should be universally enforced, and that it does not rest with the individual sister to sanction or to permit any exception to them. If it appears to her desirable that any favour involving an exception to the general rule should occasionally be granted, it is best for the sister to ascertain the particulars from her wardmaid, and promise to ask for the required permission, or to give the necessary explanation for her. In this way order will be maintained, and the sister's authority rather strengthened than diminished. It is obvious that the decision will usually be guided by the sister's wishes; and in some cases when she may not think the request altogether reasonable, and yet hardly cares to take the responsibility of refusing it, it is pleasanter to have the definite refusal come from the final authority. Again, there are clear definitions to be observed throughout the building as to what work forms a portion of a wardmaid's duties, and what has been allotted to nurses, and to this *no exception must be made.*

It is not desirable for wardmaids and members of the nursing staff to be on terms of familiarity. Their work is of a totally different character. It leads to gossip, and it is otherwise objectionable for wardmaids and nurses or probationers to be seen taking stray meals together in the wards or scullery. Directly the sister perceives any tendency to intimacies of this kind she should promptly check it. They may help each other occasionally from motives of good-nature, but that is another question. In the ordinary course of things it is not a proceeding to be altogether encouraged, partly because they each have enough

3

to do, and partly because it has a tendency to lead to misunderstandings.

In the regular arrangement of the work the duties that have been assigned to any one set of workers must not be apportioned to another. It is for the sister to ascertain what the distinctions are and to see that they are observed. Any failure to do this creates discontent either amongst her own subordinates or in other wards, where endless discussions as to what is "fair" and what is "not fair" take place. It is a pity for a sister to weaken her position by an attempt to enforce anything contrary to the general regulations, whether she does so from ignorance or with the idea that she is at liberty to set them aside. Eventually it is certain to be a matter of complaint, and will then have to be remedied. If sisters thought more of the many ways in which the work of a whole hospital is affected by their individual management or mismanagement, they would be more ready to *ask* what was considered desirable in these and similar matters, and less inclined to risk unnecessary mistakes, than is frequently the case.

But with such points as I have mentioned, broadly defined, the remainder of the wardmaid's list of work may be filled in in accordance with the sister's own design. *How, when,* and in some details *where,* the work of a wardmaid is to be done is best arranged by the respective sisters. A full list of what the sister expects, both of the regular daily work and the special duties apportioned to each day, with the times by which the various items are to be done, should be *clearly written* and placed up in the scullery, where it will serve as a guide to the wardmaid and a convenient reminder to the sister, who has much else to think about besides. It will also be useful evidence that orders have previously been given, and probably understood, if any neglect suggests the excuse that this is not the case. Although the individual wardmaid will soon learn the regular routine " by heart," a clean copy should always be in its place. The value of this arrangement will be quickly experienced any day when the wardmaid does not come, and a substitute who is possibly altogether strange to the ward, if not to the hospital, appears in her stead. What can be more annoying for a sister, who is perhaps busy with anxious cases, than to prove the value of her own wardmaid by the inconvenience of suddenly finding every little detail of her work left untouched, which means that something is wrong in every direction ? The routine so familiar to the usual worker is a mystery to the stranger, even if she be a capable person, and she will need to be told every few minutes what to do next. If there is a detailed list placed where all can read it, matters will be considerably simplified. Any nurse or probationer will be able to give the necessary instructions, the work will be accomplished with less delay, and the difficulty minimised for the sister, and indeed for every one concerned.

Hospital sisters should always arrange their work with a view to meeting emergencies with as little confusion as possible, and when these arise they must endeavour to keep their minds free to judge of the *relative* importance of the conflicting claims which are pressing upon them. For instance, a dying patient needing and perhaps asking for "sister" cannot be neglected or refused because "no one has begun to clean the grates," though it may be long past the hour at which all traces of such work would usually be cleared away ; yet, on the other hand, *the grates must be cleaned.* The question is, how can a sister secure that these matters shall be properly managed, not only in the ordinary course of events, but when difficulties suddenly arise ? The troubles of a hospital sister are like those of the rest of the world, inasmuch as "they never come singly". The day that the wardmaid fails it may probably happen that one of the staff nurses is not well enough to come on duty, and the substitute, in the very desire to do the best possible for the patients, will be obliged to ask sister a number of questions, every one of which would probably have been unnecessary in ordinary circumstances.

In the meantime there will doubtless be several cases requiring sister's special attention, for that is the normal state of affairs amongst every set of fifty or sixty patients. None of these complications could have been foreseen or prevented. The supply of extra hands to meet the deficiency is all the help that can be given, but the utility of these, while undeniable, is often less valuable than it may appear, because, for the moment, however competent, substitutes are frequently new to the particular work that is required

of them. Such a combination of transient misfortunes
is by no means a very exceptional occurrence, though
let us hope that no sister will be unlucky enough to
have a repetition of them in her wards until she has
had a comparatively peaceful interval. But it is
exactly because these unwelcome incidents occur
unexpectedly, that it is absolutely essential to have
work so arranged that what is the duty of one person
can be taken up by a substitute with the least possible
confusion and delay. To secure this every facility
must be given to the regular workers to understand
what the routine work is, and nothing furthers this
end more systematically than a methodically kept
list of what we may conveniently term the household
work. It is necessary that this list should be altered
in conformity with what is found best in practice, if
any change has been permitted since the sister drew
it up. I have sometimes observed that sisters have
not thought it worth while to do this. Leaving up
an incorrect statement of their wishes is inconsistent
with the object of making the list at all. I may add
that there is not the least occasion for the sister to
write out clean copies of the list herself, provided she
sees that it is correctly done. There will be plenty
of willing hands to do it nicely for her, and a good
manager will save herself all superfluous trouble, if
she has learnt the true value of her time. This plan
of placing it within the power of any of her usual
subordinates to give the needed instructions for
household work to any new-comer, who may be
sent to the wards in an emergency, is all that any

sister can do towards making the best of the un-
toward circumstances, unless we add the additional
help that all will derive from the sister's calm manner
and unruffled temper on such·occasions.

A sister cannot give her attention to everything at
once, but if she has thoroughly mastered the details
of all that she has to manage, she will be able to
make a little extra attention to the matter which
presses at the moment very effectual, more especially
if she takes care that most of those working with her
are familiar with her wishes. If this is the case, they
are almost certain to be ready to forward them. The
daily inspection of the wardmaid's work, the condition of the refrigerator, the milk and beer cans, the
scullery, lavatory, etc., will take very little time. A
glance, as the sister gains experience, will be sufficient to show her whether all is as it should be, but
directly she fails to display some manifestation of
interest in that department of the work it will
deteriorate. It is an error for her to suppose that
because she always finds these matters fairly straight
they will therefore remain so without her attention,
and she must not lose sight of the fact that her
inspection, and the praise that, we may hope, she
may occasionally find reason to bestow, are chiefly
instrumental in producing the desired result.

The sister must also display interest in the scrubbing of floors, if she wishes it well done, for few
people do their best, whatever their work may be,
if their efforts are habitually ignored. A slight
evidence of continuous interest on the part of the

sister is all that is required. The good workers will readily respond to this ; those who do not should, in kindness and justice, have a little more vigorous supervision for a time, but such women as will only work under the stimulus of perpetual fault-finding are seldom worth retaining. A sister's time and temper are too valuable to be expended in fruitless efforts to get her wards properly scrubbed. She must obtain this result, but she should be enabled to do this by giving the matter a *due*, not an *undue* share of her attention.

The same thoughtful observation that secures the general cleanliness will note such repairs as are constantly needed throughout these large wards. Handles will come off doors, windows need mending, ventilators will refuse to open or shut from time to time, and sundry requirements of a similar nature will have to be reported in the right direction to procure their prompt repair. A sister should teach the nurses in charge of their respective wards to call her attention to these matters, and blame them if they leave the sole responsibility of noticing these defects to her, but eventually it rests with the sister to see that they are speedily remedied.

All articles in the wards, from bedsteads and chairs to kettles and teapots and brushes and brooms, must be kept in good condition and in the right place. The sister should see that all these things are used with proper care and economy, and should never procure an order for any portion of the stock to be replenished without having the condemned article

brought for her inspection. There will be no difficulty in observing this simple rule if the orders are
not left to be written at the last moment, and no
attempts to evade it will be made by nurses or
wardmaids, if it is pleasantly and invariably enforced
by the sister. Whether a single broom or scrubbing
brush would serve for another week or two would be
a very trivial question, but the whole principle of
economy in these matters is by no means trivial in
any item of expenditure necessary for the working
of a large institution. Everything should be kept in
good condition for use, with the freedom from waste
and extravagance on the one hand, and slovenliness
on the other, which would prevail in a well-ordered
household. To permit the hospital property to be
used unfairly, either in the attempt to be so econo-
mical with the implements that the work cannot be
properly done, or from a tendency to be too extrava-
gant, is a carelessness on the part of the responsible
person that can scarcely be considered conscientious.
It need hardly be said that the inclination to extravagance is the much more general failing, but I have
known sisters who, with the best intentions, have
erred in the opposite direction, and lost sight of the
fact that their duty is to maintain *everything* in efficient working order. The sister who is a good house-
keeper will find none of the requisites for cleaning
beneath her attention. If she does not take the
trouble to look up materials that will do for floor-
cloths, etc., she may be sure that something will be
used for the purpose; probably lint, cotton wool, or

other articles of considerable value as compared to those well adapted for these domestic uses, will be seized upon if nothing else is at hand. I have myself seen a nurse catch up a piece of good, clean cotton wool to wipe away some dust; and although no amount of supervision will entirely prevent careless nurses from culpable wastefulness, it certainly rests with the sister to leave them no shadow of an excuse for it, by providing a sufficient and proper supply of suitable materials for all general cleaning purposes. Each sister can only act to the best of her judgment and learn by experience, but the point that I would insist on is that she *must* use her own judgment, and not get into an easy-going, good-natured way of taking it for granted that old things are worn out and new things are wanted, without seeing for herself that this is the case.

The ventilation of the wards, including as it does the condition of fires and windows, has a perpetual claim upon the sister's attention. Her object is that this shall always be the best possible consistent with circumstances. To ensure this she must educate the nurses in charge of each ward to a sense of individual responsibility in the matter, and not allow them to depend solely upon her. It is true that she can help them materially, and that as she passes from one ward to another she has a better opportunity for noticing the comparative freshness of the atmosphere than the nurse, who may probably have been working in it for some time; but if the sister's observation is quick and her management of the nurses good, they will soon respond to encouraging treatment, and be anxious that she shall find no cause for complaint. The ventilation of wards is by no means an easy matter, even when every appliance to enable a good result has been provided. Many patients are great enemies to fresh air. They have a conviction that an open window will do them a serious injury, and a good deal of tact is occasionally needed to persuade them to the contrary. If we reflect on the crowded homes from which the majority of our patients come, we shall understand that the prejudice is not altogether as unreasonable from their point of view as it appears to us, and whilst insisting upon the proper ventilation of the ward, the sister should impress upon her nurses the necessity of protecting every patient from draught, and of showing a due regard to their individual comfort. Patients will often grumble at a nurse, and submit without a murmur to the very same arrangement if it is sister's wish. She will be wise to utilise this fact, without giving any evidence that she is aware of it, to soften the tendency to friction between nurses and patients which sometimes exists, irrespective of any fault on the part of a nurse. When there is complete understanding between sister and nurse, and both are earnestly uniting their efforts for the comfort and welfare of the patients, it is wonderful how simply the little difficulties that arise are overcome. A nurse may see that it is best to yield to the angry and perhaps unreasonable protests of a patient who, in hospital phraseology, is "inclined to be troublesome," and refrain for the time from opening a window that, for the due ventilation of the ward, should not long remain shut. She may tell sister privately that "No. 10" grumbles at the prospect of having such and such a window opened, though for various reasons it is desirable. If when sister comes into the ward she goes over and opens the said window herself, observing, "I think, nurse, this window should be open," and the nurse has the discretion to let the matter pass with a quiet "Yes, sister," in nine cases out of ten the patient will submit without a word, and feel secretly grateful to nurse for not repeating to sister his recent protest that it will give him "his death of cold!" This is merely a trifling illustration of how much may be achieved by a little forbearance and tact towards those whose condition should lead us to give it *to*, rather than to exact it *from* them. I am frequently led to attach much value to these unselfish qualities, by the painful evidence of their absence in some of the trifling disturbances that arise between good earnest workers, and the recipients of their care. It is in such small matters as the opening of a window, or the shutting of a door, that a little more consideration towards those who are in the wrong would avert the difficulty. If a sister never looks at the ward thermometer herself, she need not expect that her nurses will do so. She should cultivate this useful habit in them by example, and by inquiries which indicate that she expects them to have ascertained more or less recently what is the exact temperature recorded.

The condition of the fires may sometimes call for remark from the sister, for she will be exceptionally fortunate in her subordinates if she does not occasionally find that, with the best intentions, some energetic person has piled the coals far up the chimney in a manner which renders it in imminent danger of catching fire. If it is not so bad as that, there is still great waste in burning coals in a position which compels nearly all the heat produced to be lost to the ward. On the other hand, it is very undesirable that fires should be kept too low, and that they should present a dismal, smouldering appearance, instead of contributing to the cheerful aspect of the ward by the bright glow which has such a pleasant effect. Everybody knows that the majority of servants have an unhappy habit of thoughtlessly making up a large fire on a warm sunny day, when it is just a question whether one's room would not be pleasanter without a fire at all, and most of us have shivered before now over a few black embers, doing duty for a fire, when the mere sight of a cheerful blaze and of the red glow suggestive of warmth would have contributed materially to our comfort. As in most of the practical matters of domestic housekeeping, a mind educated in these subjects is needed to guide the acting hands. The importance of efficiency in such details is enhanced rather than diminished in a hospital, because they influence the comfort and welfare of the sick.

The light of a ward needs but little attention as compared to the warmth. Every ray of sunshine is welcome, except when it pours down too strongly upon a patient's bed, or when any light is obviously too dazzling for a patient's eyes. In either case an observant nurse will speedily remedy the discomfort. A sister should not fail to do this if it has been left for her to notice, but she should teach the nurse that it was her duty to have noticed and paid attention to this detail, without needing a reminder on the subject from sister.

In all these matters a sister should hold herself ultimately but not directly responsible, and she should lose no opportunity of giving her assistants a clear view of their individual and mutual responsibilities. It is but fair to them that their own powers of observation should be trained, and that they should thus gain the full value of their practical experience. This they can never do if they are accustomed to depend upon sister in the every-day matters about which they should learn to judge for themselves. If a sister encourages this dependence upon herself, either from a reprehensible sense of self-importance, or from a want of power to elicit the best of which other characters are capable, the work as a whole cannot fail to suffer from her deficiency in this respect. Yet, it is obvious, that while subordinates are acquiring the knowledge of their various duties, their defects must be supplied by the sister, so that no confusion or ignorance may mar the efficiency of the work that each day brings. To be able to work well without supervision is to be an invaluable helper, and gives proof of having gained a certain standpoint in one's profession as a nurse.

But, to be able to supervise others is a further stage of development, calling for the exercise of greater powers. That it is easier to do a familiar thing oneself than to show another person how to do it is a mere truism, but it is the latter and more difficult task that a sister must accept.

To encourage others to think and act for themselves, whilst ensuring the efficiency of the work for which she is responsible, by supplying their defects, is the real object at which a sister should aim. That this is comparatively little realised by some, the nature of their achievements will show, but those who accept this as one of their guiding principles will testify, without hesitation, that it lightens their own work on the whole, while it ensures a more successful and more permanent result. The same kind of supervision from the sister which is instrumental in securing well-regulated warmth and ventilation, will promote general order and neatness in other details. Practical matters claim attention first, but this can be given without disregarding those arrangements which, if not absolutely essential, are greatly conducive to the welfare and comfort of those whose home is the ward for the time while they are living in it. The nurse who has the most taste will be encouraged to display it by the sister's appreciation. The one who is least gifted with the feminine knack of giving those finishing touches to the arrangement of the surroundings which impart a feeling of " homeliness " to the whole, will be eager to do her best if only " to please sister," and will gradually learn in this way to attach due importance to what, it may be, she has previously ignored. A withered flower will be banished as quickly as dust from a ward where it is certain that "sister" will notice it at once, and fresh flowers will be eagerly welcomed and tastefully disposed of when it is known that "sister" will greet their appearance with prompt recognition and pleasure.

These are only a few of the "little things" by which a thoughtful person will contribute to the pleasing effect which cheerful surroundings have upon us all. Sick people are doubly susceptible of these influences, because in their depressed condition they are more dependent upon them, and beyond the reach of those changes which tend to direct the current of their thoughts into more hopeful channels. It is true that we are appreciative of beauty in very varied degrees, and that if we expect any marked results from our care for trifles, we shall be disappointed; but those who have turned their attention most to these matters will be aware that many, who are not conscious that they are deriving any pleasure, much less any good, from their immediate surroundings, are, all the while, *unconsciously* responding to their influence. Everything that helps to brighten the aspect of a ward in a hospital should be cordially welcomed by those who have anything to do with its management.

I must not conclude this chapter without reference to one or two other matters to which it is essential that the sister's attention should daily be directed, but their very importance makes it less likely that they would be overlooked than some of the smaller things I have mentioned.

The quality and condition of the food provided for the patients, and the manner in which it is served, is a matter about which a sister should be extremely particular. In all probability it will be impossible, even if it were desirable in such large wards, that she should see to the distribution of every diet herself. But it is a distinct duty for her to examine every article of diet that is sent into her wards, that she may be in a position to fill up the daily food report in a perfectly accurate manner. The sister should be able to answer definitely any questions that may arise as to the quality of any food that is supplied. Some sisters are more careless about this than they probably would be if they realised fully how greatly patients are dependent upon their care and attention, in a matter which, in many cases, forms an important part of the treatment that the doctor desires them to receive. Sisters will soon learn by daily experience to distinguish between defects in the food itself, or the manner of preparation, and such as patients with no appetite may imagine to exist. In every case it is obviously the sister's duty to fill up the paper which she signs *exactly in accordance with her own judgment* on every item referred to in the report. A sister must divide her attention between observation of the quality of the food and the proper distribution of diets, and must see that each patient receives his dinner in an appetising form. She should pass round the wards for the purpose of noting the manner in which the dinners are being served by the nurses and probationers. Unless the sister takes this interest, thorough efficiency will not be maintained. Dinners will get cold while the patient is waiting for a knife and fork. A plate may be in an impossible position, and the patient lie looking at a dinner that is getting cold, until his uncertain appetite has quite turned against the food that he might have eaten, had it been quickly and invitingly served. Again, a patient may be able to feed himself—a much more appetising process than being fed—and yet be unable to cut up the dinner, or reach anything that is not placed close at hand. It is for staff nurses and probationers to attend to these details, but the training which attaches due importance to them is a very gradual process, and constant supervision is required to ensure that these *little* matters, so essential to the comfort of patients, are not overlooked.

The sister must see that the stimulants are duly distributed and administered in compliance with the orders received. She must arrange for this to be efficiently done, and take care that the least possible time elapses between the arrival of the supply of stimulants in the ward and their careful measurement and distribution into the separate bottles allotted to those patients who are " on " stimulants. The sister must take care that her attention is immediately called to any mistake, or apparent mistake, in the quantity sent up, so that

4

she may be able to take the proper responsibility of getting it rectified. Provided that this is done, there is no necessity for the sister to undertake the daily measurements herself, as this, like other purely mechanical, though by no means unimportant duties, should be given into subordinate, but thoroughly reliable hands.

The care of the strong poisons that are used in the wards is a matter of the gravest responsibility. The point to which the sister must direct unceasing attention, besides seeing that the labels are clean, correct, and legible, is having every poison locked up the moment that the bottles or jars containing them are no longer required. If they are allowed to be left about until other matters are attended to, great and unnecessary risk is attached to the proceeding. There is the twofold fear that nurses may use these poisons in mistake for other things, and that patients may get possession of them and swallow them, accidentally or otherwise. In either case the result is too appalling to be calmly contemplated, even as a remote possibility, and the mere thought of so terrible a contingency should suffice to promote unceasing care on the part of the sister, and stimulate her to untiring efforts to impress all who work in her wards with the extreme importance of this duty. She should take pains to explain to each one exactly where the poisons are kept and her rule concerning them. The first time that she finds it has been disregarded, she must speak very seriously to the delinquent, giving her to understand that it will be her duty as sister to report the negligence if it occurs again. The sister will be gravely to blame herself if, in the event of a second failure to render exact obedience in so important a matter, she does not carry out her expressed intention. We all know that accidents will happen, and in many cases it is well to take a lenient view of faults that have been inadvertently committed; but carelessness, that may so easily lead to such terrible results, is not a matter to be casually overlooked, either for the sake of the unthinking individual, who may yet learn better, or for the welfare of others. Nothing but unremitting attention, and a consistently good example on the part of the sister, will meet the requirements of the case. She would do well to remember that while she is looking after her own wards in this important particular, she is helping to form habits of carefulness in those who are working under her, for which they may have reason to be filled with gratitude in the future of their work.

The charge of the ward-linen demands a share of attention, although it is a much less anxious matter than that to which I have just referred. The sister should take care that nothing is put back into the linen cupboard when it returns from the laundry until it has been duly looked over, and if this point is strictly adhered to, the other details are secured with but little trouble. There are three objects in looking it over : to see that the numbers have been correctly returned, that nothing belonging to other wards has been placed in this collection—a very pardonable

error now and again when such large assortments
have to be made—and to see that such articles as
require mending are separated from those which are
to be used next. Perhaps I should have said that
four objects were to be borne in mind, and included
the thorough airing of linen, for this is a point of
paramount importance, and one that will never be
overlooked by a good sister, in connection with its
examination on return from the laundry.

There is need for judicious management in regulating the supply of linen, to avoid the extremes of too
great economy to be consistent with the needs of the
patients and the cleanliness of the wards, and of the
extravagance which needlessly increases the heavy
amount of washing to be done in a large hospital.
Judgment is necessary as to the kind as well
as the amount of linen to be allotted to different
cases. It is evidence of very thoughtless management for a sister to give out sheets, blankets,
etc., without any regard to the character of the
cases for which they may be required. Cases of
burns and skin diseases, for instance, where the
remedies applied may be of a very greasy nature, are
more than ordinarily likely to stain and otherwise de-
stroy the bedding with which they come in contact,
and should not have the newest linen allotted to
them, but these things should be distributed with
care and discrimination. It ought not to be necessary to point out the desirability of what is simply
common-sense in such a matter, but the thoughtless-
ness frequently displayed in regard to it suggests

some comment on the subject. The want of care
in reference to repairs leads to a wasteful manner of
dealing with hospital property, that, as I have previously observed, is not consistent with the work of
a conscientious sister. For the most part sisters
cannot well manage to secure that their own mending should be done in their own busy wards.
When they have patients able and willing to attend
to it so much the better, but when this is not the
case, the sister can at least see that articles needing
repair are sent to the linen room for this purpose,
and are not used again and sent to the laundry
before they have received the necessary attention.

The manner in which the ward-linen is cared for,
or neglected, usually manifests itself clearly when
the appointed time for taking the inventory arrives.
Not only is the carefulness, or the carelessness of
the ward sister shown by the accuracy of the
numbers on her list and the condition of the linen
displayed, but the manner in which her preparations
for the inventory-taking have been made, will go far
to indicate her method or the want of it in dealing
with this matter. It is needless to say that the ward
sister should have carefully counted over everything
with her nurses, before going through the official inspection with the matron or the matron's represent-
ative. She should be perfectly aware of her losses
(if any) beforehand, and not wait for the inspector to
point them out to her, with the inevitable necessity
of counting the articles in question all over again to
ascertain that no error in the counting has arisen.

By so doing a sister not only demonstrates her own inefficiency, but, by causing this repetition, wastes time that is certainly not less valuable than her own. Sheets, blankets, etc., which are actually in use on beds at the time, should have their marks all arranged at one corner for this occasion, so that they may be easily seen, and other articles shown up with similar facility for examining them. A methodically prepared inventory should be a lesson on this particular detail to every nurse and probationer working in the set of wards in question, besides serving as an indication of a sister's powers of general management.

The mattresses need inspection as well as the rest of the bedding, and a sister should be particular in looking after her nurses on this point. She must insist upon the judicious use of mackintoshes, and remember that economy in this respect is a secondary consideration, while soiling the mattresses is a comparatively expensive process, and allowing these to be spoiled, by having no mackintosh to protect them in accident or other cases, is not a justifiable use of hospital property. In all these matters the sister's influence will exercise an effect in exact accordance with the manner in which it is exerted. She must bend all her energies to secure a uniformly good result in connection with all the details of domestic management that I have enumerated, and in the many others that will doubtless occur to her in the midst of her daily work. She must clearly realise that what she can actually do with her own hands is very little—a mere nothing as compared with all that has to be accomplished in any one particular even in her own wards,—and that while her hands are always ready to help in every direction, it is for her to keep them free for this purpose. Her main business is to secure that all these matters are efficiently attended to by those whose duty it is.

A sister " takes her place " in the ward by manifesting an interest in everything that has to be done, with the object of ensuring that there will be no neglect in the management of these essentials when her attention is called off in other legitimate directions. The sister who can feel a well-grounded confidence that everything has gone on in her wards with perfect regularity and precision, when unexpected claims have prevented her giving the usual attention to them, is to be congratulated upon so satisfactory a result. She has evidently found the right method of securing the favourable conditions that are as essential for the patients in her absence as in her presence. The sister who cannot be absent for a few hours, without universal discomfort ensuing, may be very hard-working, but she has achieved much less, and had better change her system of management as soon as possible. To sum up my meaning in a very homely simile, if a sister looks upon the wards as a clock and herself as the key, after seeing that the works are in good order she will *wind it up regularly*, and be able to leave it for a time in confidence that it will go well. No one will say that the key is of no consequence, because the clock does its work steadily, but rather that it is well regulated and never allowed to run down.

CHAPTER III.

IT appears to me that considerable misunderstanding prevails, or perhaps it would be more accurate to say that there is a distinct want of understanding, as to the relationship of sisters and their staff nurses. It will be remembered that my remarks are addressed to those who have charge of such large wards, that their office virtually becomes that of superintendent of the nursing of a certain number of patients, rather than what we conceive to be the work of a head nurse in a smaller department. In hospitals where fewer beds are placed under the charge of each sister, the distinctions between the work of a sister or a head nurse and her assistants are much less marked. In that case the sister's work involves less supervision and more actual nursing, and there will consequently be less difficulty in finding women capable of filling such posts. The same need for conscientious workers with a thorough knowledge of nursing exists in both cases, but in the one instance it is not necessary to possess much administrative power to ensure success.

For women lacking this greater power of being able to direct others, and therefore unfitted for the larger responsibility, there is almost unlimited scope for the happy exercise of their full powers in the office of staff nurse in a large hospital, or that of head nurse in smaller hospitals, as in many respects the duties of the two offices are similar. The best preparation for a sister's post, whether on a large or a small scale, is undoubtedly the experience that can be gained as a staff nurse. All the knowledge acquired in that capacity is essential to the satisfactory fulfilment of the duties of the higher grade. But there can be no question that the value of the experience gained by any staff nurse will mainly depend upon the sister under whom she is working. It is therefore important to staff nurses individually, as well as to the sister and the working of the institution as a whole, that their mutual relationship be clearly defined and well understood.

It must not be supposed, because I avoid all reference to the details of nursing itself, that I am inclined to underrate their importance, for such is by no means the case. It is only that at present I am thinking of and speaking to trained nurses, whether acting as sisters or in less responsible posts. These, whilst profiting by the renewed opportunities for gaining fresh experience which hospital life affords, have yet acquired the general and rudimentary knowledge of nursing which forms an essential qualification for the position in which they have been placed.

Some sisters appear to find it very difficult to know how much or how little it is well to leave to their staff nurses. This uncertainty is naturally

reflected upon the staff nurses themselves, and it
will be found that they entertain their own views —
very erroneous ones for the most part, as they would
soon see for themselves in the light of a fuller experience—as to what their position is or ought to be.
Their view of a sister's merits will generally turn
on the question as to how much she "interferes"
with them, and how far she "trusts" them.   Both
expressions are suggestive to me of the mistaken ideas
that are prevalent as to their mutual responsibilities.

If the simple question were asked any nurse, she
would unhesitatingly admit that sister was the head
of the ward.   She will " ask sister " readily enough
about those matters that she thinks come within her
province, and indeed is thankful that " sister " is there
to be asked, when it is a question which involves any
responsibility that she is reluctant to take upon herself.   But many a nurse in speaking without reserve
to one of her fellow-workers would be heard to declare
with more or less emphasis that " sister *has no
business* to interfere " with this, that and the other,
or " I am quite miserable with sister ; she doesn't
trust me a bit, but looks into everything herself ".
If a sister is responsible for everything in her wards,
obviously everything *is* her business, and any inclination on the part of her subordinates to call this in
question must either arise from the *manner* in which
she has interfered, or from a tendency to what is
familiarly known as " uppishness " on the part of the
nurse, and that cannot be approved or permitted, as it
is subversive of order, and can scarcely arise from any

laudable quality in the nurse's character. In dealing with nurses of this type it is better for the sister to persist in the course that she thinks right, even if she gains a temporary reputation of being a "regular fidget," or of "giving one no peace," than it is for her to yield to the opinions of her subordinates in such matters. If she is gentle and consistent, she will carry her point and win her nurses at the same time. Probably both sisters and nurses are to blame when such feelings arise, but the larger share of blame surely rests with the sisters, inasmuch as it is for them to perceive the necessity of infusing a different spirit into their workers, and if all were agreed at this moment that improvement were desirable, it would yet remain for individual sisters to introduce it.

It is a great temptation to busy sisters of large wards, to let sundry details of the management drift entirely into other hands, and the result is much confusion that might otherwise be avoided, and too frequently grave injustice to probationers, of which, however, I shall have more to say hereafter. On the other hand, sisters whose idea of fulfilling their duty consists in doing everything themselves, and who cannot learn to delegate work to others, keeping themselves free for the performance of such things as may be more strictly characterised as sisters' work, are practically unfitted for the management of large wards. This failing mars the achievements of so many earnest and otherwise capable workers that, I am inclined to think, it is one that all women in taking up public work should specially guard them-

selves against. It originates in praiseworthy motives,
and is consequently the more difficult to find fault
with in others, and to detect in ourselves. Nevertheless it is to be gravely deplored as a weakness
which places a distinct limitation upon our powers
of usefulness.

The leading idea that a sister should instil into the
minds of her staff nurses, and which she should
constantly keep fresh in her own mind in her dealings
with them, is that of co-operation towards a common
object, *i.e.*, the comfort and welfare of the patients,
and the orderly performance of such duties as apper-
tain to their respective offices, in a manner that is due
to the hospital in which and for which they are both
working. The idea of co-operation, which is simple
to grasp and yet comparatively little realised, is more
effectual in banishing the petty rivalry which is ever
likely to arise, and, yet, always sadly out of place,
between hospital workers, than any other principle
of universal application in this matter. It helps to
sink the idea of "self," which is generally the cause
of these injured feelings. The mere thought of the
work for which both sister and nurse are probably
anxious to do their best, and which can but suffer
from any want of harmony between them, will act as
a wholesome check upon those personal feelings that
are such a hindrance to the performance of good work.
The problem that a sister has to solve for her own
guidance in managing staff nurses is, how to combine
the supervision which her office demands of her, with
the confidence that will inspire them to do their

utmost, and to produce the best results of which they are individually capable.

A feeling of mutual confidence is the only basis for harmonious work that can be relied upon. The sister need think no time wasted that goes towards creating or establishing this feeling between herself and every individual worker with whom she is brought into personal contact. Where this feeling mutually exists the rest will be comparatively easy; where it does not many difficulties will inevitably occur, and no pains must be spared to cultivate it. It is impossible to prevent all misunderstandings between workers of various tempers and temperaments, under circumstances that are, occasionally, very trying to both, but it is probable that the number of these misunderstandings will be diminished, if we see in which direction they are likely to occur, and there is a cordial desire to avoid them.

The sister must treat her nurses with confidence as a matter of course, not as a special favour, and regard it as simply out of the question that anything she says or does concerning their work or the patients, *could* be misinterpreted as implying any distrust. If trustworthy nurses, who have not been accustomed to this wise method of treatment, are inclined to misunderstand and resent it at first, they will soon learn to like it when they feel sure that no doubt of them is felt or intended; and if those who are not trustworthy dislike it, that is but an additional proof that it is a wise system which tends to eliminate unsatisfactory workers. If a sister does *not* trust a

nurse, the sooner she finds an opportunity of telling
her so, and explaining her reason for the want of
confidence, the better. The mere fact of being greeted
with a candid statement of this kind will inspire the
nurse with an ·unmistakable conviction that she is
dealing with a straightforward person, and one who
is anxious to be fair to her and just towards the work
at the same time. If the want of confidence has
arisen from a misunderstanding of circumstances, the
nurse has a good opportunity for putting the matter
straight, and clearing away the wrong impression
which the sister may not unreasonably have formed
concerning her. If this is not possible, it will be
wholesome for the nurse to know that she is understood and valued accordingly.

In work of all sorts it is often necessary to put up
with workers that are very far removed from the
best. That the work suffers from their deficiencies
is obvious, but it remains for us, as far as possible,
to bring out the best of which each one is capable
so long as they are the material with which our work
has to be done. In those cases where mutual respect
and confidence are impossible, the highest results
cannot be attained, and it is idle to expect them.

The sister's supervision should take the form of
active *interest* in all that goes on in her wards, and in
every duty which falls to the share of each one of her
workers. If this is the case, they will eagerly turn to
her for help, sympathy, and appreciation in all they
do. The question of "whose business" this is will
be completely submerged in the desire to perform

every item of their work, not without sister's knowledge or "interference," but in the exact manner
that sister will approve. The wish to be a valuable
helper, by *thoroughness* in the performance of every
duty, is infinitely more inspiring than the wish to be
"let alone," and " to be allowed to do my own work
in my own way," which some staff nurses conceive
to be the chief duty of a sister towards them. In
this narrow view they quite lose sight of the fact that
this is not consistent with the sister's own duty, and
that it cannot be the best thing for them either. Yet
I would be slow to blame staff nurses for not per-
ceiving this if there are sisters who have not yet
discovered it themselves.

How many have made inefficient sisters, failed to
maintain discipline in their wards, and to exercise
due control over their subordinates, by not realising
their own responsibilities and feebly resigning them
into other hands ! And this, not with any intention
of shirking their duty, but with a sort of ill-defined
idea that, as they cannot *do* everything themselves,
they will spare themselves trouble, and please the
nurses, by leaving everything to them, when they
have once given some evidence that they can be de-
pended upon. Results have shown in innumerable
instances the folly of such proceedings. If a sister
deliberately set herself to limit her own power, could
she find a more effectual plan for so doing than by
thus lessening the possibilities of her usefulness?
If the nurses may not look to her for that daily
appreciation of their work, and that sympathy with

their many difficulties which the best workers need
to encourage them, to whom shall they look for it?
Surely no sister, who sees where she is drifting by
refusing to take her proper share of responsibility,
would willingly adopt a system that will ultimately
lead to her wishes being practically, if not intention-
ally, ignored. A sister should let her nurses' work
be clearly defined, should let them be responsible to
her for the exact and punctual fulfilment of every
detail, should make a point of leaving the actual
performance of almost all that has to be done to
them, so that all could go on smoothly for a while
without her, but she must manifest a continuous
interest in it all, and insist that she is kept duly
informed of all that takes place.

Once again, we cannot do better than regard the
set of wards as a united family of which sister is the
head. Her interest in all is assumed as a matter of
course. No one would think of ignoring or defying
her wishes, though they would gladly turn to her
for help in a difficulty. Each one is free to follow
her own duties, with due regard to the convenience
of the whole, this being regulated by the one who is
responsible for the well-being of all, and therefore
best able to judge how that may be combined with
individual freedom. This illustration appears to me
useful as a practical guide to the general principle
that is most likely to produce universally beneficial
results.

The sister is responsible for seeing that all her
subordinates, *as well as she herself*, obey the general

rules allotted to them by the hospital, and she will accomplish this with least trouble and at the same time most effectually by *expecting* each one to carry them out as a matter of course. Her supervision can in many respects be combined with the ordinary courtesies of life. To dispense with the good-morning and good-night greeting, customary in daily intercourse, is always a mistake. There is no reason why the due observance of what it would be considered a rudeness to omit in the family should not serve for the "reporting" which is essential to the maintenance of punctuality in the wards. I do not mean to imply that no workers would be exact with regard to time and in the performance of their duties if they were left entirely to themselves, but, taking the average type of humanity with which we have to deal, we must admit that laxity in these respects is very apt to occur ; and, in order to avoid invidious distinctions between individual workers and to ensure the best result throughout, some system of supervision is necessary. That which is secured under the guise of the daily courtesies of life is obviously preferable and not less efficient.

As London Hospital sisters are not on duty until 8 A.M. and day staff nurses and probationers are due in their wards at 7 A.M., the sister should arrange that one of her dependable night staff nurses should mark the punctual or unpunctual attendance of all working in that set of wards, in a small book kept for the purpose, and placed ready for sister's inspection when she first comes on duty.

5

Experience proves that the fact of the whole day nursing staff being registered as to attendance at breakfast in the nursing home, does not necessarily ensure the punctual arrival of each individual worker at the post allotted to her, so that this must be systematically secured. If any one is late, it is easy for the sister to ask for the explanation when she comes on duty, and the fact that the sister *knows* exactly what takes place is the safeguard against irregularities.

It is most unsatisfactory when an inquiry is made about some nurse or probationer who may not be on duty, or some one who may have received orders to present themselves in that particular ward that morning, if the sister is obliged to confess that she has not missed them in the one case, or has not been told of the fresh arrival in the other.

Knowledge of all that goes on in a large ward implies power in the sister, and certainly places power in her hands. It can only be obtained, when there are a number of subordinates, by a system which induces it, and makes the want of it obvious. Punctuality in the going off and coming on duty at other times is secured by the sister exacting a simple statement of the fact from each of her nurses, and if the idea of mistrust has been mutually dismissed, no shade of irritation will be associated with the only method that enables both to do their duty.

Again, with regard to the nursing of the patients. It falls to the staff nurses' share for the most part to execute the doctor's orders. It is they who make and apply poultices, etc., etc., though the sister is ultimately responsible to the doctor for seeing that his orders are carried out. But how is the sister to fulfil this responsibility if she is simply to take it for granted that everything has been properly attended to without ascertaining that this is the case?

If a staff nurse leaves it for sister to inquire whether each detail has received attention, that is throwing the burden of remembering entirely upon the sister, and unduly taxing her powers. The staff nurse should make a point of telling sister distinctly that such and such things have been done for such and such patients, and until she has acquired this habit, the sister should insist upon questioning her, and upon seeing that the various details have been carried out. The important fact for the sister is to educate the staff nurses into this useful custom. It will prove helpful to the latter, because it will give them a reason for thoughtfully summing up the orders given for different patients, with a view of being able to report to sister that various items have been duly attended to. Their memory will be rather improved than otherwise by this method; it will prove an excellent check upon less careful workers, and it will enable sister to remind them of what may be left undone. Even those who are less conscientious would hesitate to report that a certain detail had been attended to if this was not the case, when they might be less scrupulous of leaving some things undone on the mere chance of sister discovering the

omission, and with the ready excuse of " I forgot "
to fall back upon.

The same applies to the patients' diet. It is for
the staff nurse to make herself acquainted with any
alterations that the doctor has made, or to mention
to sister any special article of food for which any
patient may have expressed a desire, to enable sister
to ascertain from the doctor if the wish may be
granted. The individual wants of sixty patients can
scarcely be attended to properly in these respects,
even at the cost of much anxiety on the part of the
sister, unless the staff nurses realise that it is their
duty to afford efficient help. The idea of co-operation
will be strengthened by this practical method of
aiding sister in the satisfactory fulfilment of the
common work. Sisters and staff nurses will soon
prove in their busy lives how much help they can
give and receive in this manner.

The rules as to the respective duties of night and
day nurses should be clearly laid down and adhered
to as far as the exigencies of the work permit. Any
help that one set of workers may like to give the
other is all very well when their respective duties are
accomplished, and within the time that the rules of
the hospital allow them to be on duty, but it is a
bad plan for one to do the work of the other, leaving
her own work undone, and such exceptions should
not be permitted.

With regard to the work of night and day
nurses ; there are certain broad distinctions that
apply to the whole hospital, and it does not rest

in the hands of individual sisters to alter these, but rather to see that their universal adoption is enforced. For instance, it is understood that every appliance is left clean and ready for the use of each set of workers when the one goes off and the other comes on duty. Night nurses are not allowed to make the beds, except, of course, when the needs of any special patient may require them to do so. The general bed-making of the ward is too heavy work for night nurses towards the expiration of their long hours on duty, and, in hospitals where it is customary for them to do this, there is an obvious risk of patients being disturbed too early with the view of the nurses " getting forward with the work ". Besides, it is the day nurses who are responsible for the beds—i.e., their comfortable and neat condition—and the making of beds should be the first work of day nurses and probationers when they come on duty in the morning. If the wards are unusually full and heavy, it should be remembered that the work that falls to the share of the night staff will be increased in proportion as well as the bed-making, and that mixing the duties of each is more likely to introduce confusion than facilitate progress with the work. Nevertheless, a heavy ward may suddenly become light by the loss of the most anxious cases, or the incessant changes which occur in the numbers of patients throughout the building, may result in an increase or diminution of nursing power in one set of wards, dependent on other claims in the hospital. When this takes

place it is within the sister's province to leave word
with her night nurse that such and such a probationer on day duty shall act as night probationer
under such and such a nurse from 7 A.M. to 9·20 A.M.
If the amount of night nursing power has become
in excess of the immediate needs, or if the supply of
day nursing power is exceptionally short through
the failure of the expected number of workers to
come on duty, the sister may equally arrange that
a certain night probationer shall act as day probationer under a certain staff nurse from 7 A.M. to
9·20 A.M.—the regular hour for all on night duty at
the London Hospital to leave the wards.   Careful
arrangement with a little foresight on the part of a
capable sister will prove invaluable.   Each one will
then have a reasonable chance of going on with the
regular work allotted to her, instead of wasting
precious moments wondering what to do next.   It
is only by judicious management in matters of this
sort that every pair of hands can be made of service,
and only by finding the work of a ward systematically organised that individual workers will grow to
perceive the value of method.   Every hospital
worker knows how much there is to be done in the
early morning, and what a busy time it is in the
wards, say from 6 A.M., the earliest hour at which
night nurses are allowed to distribute the patients'
breakfasts, until 9·30 A.M., when the wards are all
straight and in readiness for the regular visits of the
doctors.   But it should not be forgotten that from 7
A.M. to 9·20 A.M. members of night and day nursing

staffs are both on duty, and if the work is heavy, there are many hands to make it light. Of course, when those on night duty have finished the share of work allotted to them, they should help the day staff in any way they can, up to the hour when their time on duty terminates.

Night nurses and probationers should not go off duty before the right time, any more than day nurses would expect to do so, neither should they be permitted to join in the lunch or extra breakfast of those on day duty. I do not mean that they should be actually prohibited from taking a cup of tea or coffee, but the last of their regular meals during the night should be taken before the patients' breakfast at 6 A.M. The habit which some night nurses are apt to adopt, of taking a regular meal of toast, bread-and-butter, bread-and-jam, and other things of this sort at eight or nine o'clock, when the night nurses' dinner is at 10 A.M., is foolish in the extreme, and one which no sister should allow to become a regular practice. It naturally deprives the tired nurses of much appetite for the substantial meal awaiting them, and which experience shows the majority of them will be inclined to take if they do not act in the thoughtless manner I describe. I mention it because I have known sisters out of good nature allow these meals to become customary, but if they reflected upon the probable effect upon the health of their nurses of substituting a succession of irregular meals for the wholesome food provided at convenient hours

for them, they would never sanction such a proceeding.

The importance of getting work done up to time
is quickly impressed upon all new-comers, and there
must be some defect in the way the work is arranged
if all that is necessary is not accomplished in the allotted hours. Considerable waste of time and labour
takes place from the fact that they do not all know
what their own work is, but under the impression
that there is a great deal to be done, they set to
work vaguely in all directions, instead of proceeding
steadily with a given duty. It rests with the sister
to impress each of her subordinates with the necessity
of working methodically, and to arrange in smaller
details what work should be apportioned to night or
day workers, so that instead of finding themselves
at a loss what to do next, when a press of work
occurs, they each have a general knowledge of what to
go on doing towards getting it all cleared up.

No sister is justified in allowing her night nurses
and probationers to remain on duty after hours without reporting the fact and stating why it was necessary
to make the exception. The same remark applies
equally to the day nurses and probationers, but they
are due at supper immediately they leave the ward,
and their late appearance there would be noticed, so
this may serve as a check. Perhaps there is also less
temptation to keep them beyond the proper time than
frequently seems to be the case with night nurses.
Many sisters, who would be more inclined to pride
themselves upon a careful observance of hospital rules

than to set them aside, seem scarcely to realise the fact that by keeping their nurses late on duty, or allowing them to remain in the wards at an hour when, in the ordinary course of things, they have no right to be there, direct sanction is given to the breaking of a regulation that has been made for *all* who fill a certain position in the hospital, and which it is, therefore, the sister's duty to see carefully enforced. If a sister means to secure obedience, she must be thoroughly consistent in her dealings with those who work under her, and set an example of unfailing obedience to rule herself. It will not do for her to make a selection from the rules, and carry out those that she may happen to approve, whilst ignoring those that may give her some little trouble to enforce, or which she may deem undesirable.

Such a plan would be alike unfair to the general work and discipline of the institution, and detrimental to her own position and influence. Moreover, the attempt to ensure the observance of some rules, whilst manifesting a neglect for others, or the fact of being particular about having them carried out at one time and being regardless of them at another, will give her subordinates an impression that the sister fails in that justice of treatment which each one may fairly claim at her hands. To them it will appear that she "makes favourites," that she finds fault at one time and overlooks a similar failing on another occasion; and though nothing may be further from her intention than to deal unjustly with any one, or to give cause for jealousy, if the manner in which she conducts

her work depends upon the sister's moods, instead
of upon well-defined principles, it cannot but produce
an unsatisfactory effect upon those who have the mis-
fortune to be placed under her.   The regulations that
are of general application are in the hands of all whom
they may concern ; consequently the failure to observe
them is patent to all.   They cannot but respect such
sisters as insist upon having all rules loyally obeyed,
and though the sisters who neglect to do this may
have a certain amount of temporary popularity on the
ground of being " easy going," they must be content
to take a much lower place in the estimation of the
best subordinates, and, indeed, of all of them.

It should be the same with staff nurses as with
wardmaids in respect of taking the general rules as a
guide for general management, and the minor duties
are a matter for individual but systematic arrangement by each sister as she may consider best adapted
for her own wards.

If the principle, or perhaps I should say the feeling
of family life were once established, it would facilitate
the harmonious working of numbers more than can
easily be conceived.   The staff nurses will be ready
enough to suggest any alterations in the arrangements
of the work for the sister's approval, and she will be
equally ready to have the suggestions tried if they
commend themselves to her judgment, provided that
all idea of staff nurses managing the wards as *they*
think best, apart from sister's wishes, has once been
entirely dismissed.   The question, " Has such and
such a thing been done for a patient ? " will no more

create a grievance or imply mistrust, than the question of " Have you remembered to write a particular note or send a particular message?" would cause annoyance from one member of a family to another, and it is worth untiring effort on the part of the sister to bring about this tone of feeling in her wards. The opportunity that a sister has for considering the welfare and comfort of her nurses is a great help towards establishing the relationship that should exist between them. It is essential that the sister should, as far as possible, make each nurse feel that she takes a personal interest in her, and nothing will be more likely to ensure a satisfactory response from the nurse, than the conviction that sister has a kindly regard for her health, her general welfare, and, as far as may be, for her recreation and pleasure. It is not likely that persons who are never considered will as a class show habitual consideration towards others ; and it is unreasonable to expect that, if nurses are never conscious that their wants and wishes receive attention, they will be unfailing in their endeavours to put the needs of their patients, and the requirements of the work, before their more personal interests.

The mental and physical strain upon hospital nurses of every rank is considerable. The tax upon a woman's sympathy, if she possesses enough to fit her for the work, is very severe, and the more recreation of the right kind that a nurse has, the better her work will be done, and the more help she will be to her patients. To say that a nurse will be less efficient when she is tired, than when she is feeling up to her work, is merely to utter a truism, and yet it is a fact which frequently appears to be overlooked. It is often impossible to give a tired nurse the rest that a sister may be quite conscious that she needs, and we all know that anxious work, such as nursing is, has often to be done under difficulties ; but if a sister is duly impressed with the fact that by lessening fatigue, whenever possible, greater efficiency will be maintained, she will turn a little more attention to this subject for herself and for her nurses. Neither must she be disheartened by the apparent indifference with which her efforts to help the nurses in this direction may probably be met. Every one who has laboured to secure benefits for any class of workers knows what a disappointment it is to find that the very persons who reap the advantage are occasionally the last to show any appreciation of what has been done for them. It is well to be prepared for this, and gain courage to persevere in the face of this difficulty by the firm conviction that the action taken is for the best. In addition to the disinclination for going out which is rather apt to become chronic with some nurses, and which arises partly from physical fatigue, and partly from the tendency which hospital work has to become all-absorbing to those who are engaged in it, there are some who are conscious that there is plenty to do, and would prefer to remain on duty instead of taking the recreation due to them. But, except in emergencies, this should never be permitted. The organisation of the work demands and ensures that the patients shall not be left without some one

at hand to attend to them, but that is for the sister
to arrange, and the nurse will learn by experience,
however reluctantly, that she is worth more to her
patients and able to get on with her work far better
when she returns from her two hours off duty, than
would have been the case if she had remained all the
time in her ward. It may be urged, on the other
hand, that there are some nurses who would be
anxious to get off duty more frequently than would
be consistent with the welfare of the patients or fair
to the other workers, and this tendency when it exists
must be firmly held in check. The spirit of sacrifice
which should be latent in all true workers must not
be ignored when the conditions of work demand its
exercise, and when this spirit becomes conspicuous
by its absence, as is sometimes the case, it becomes
the duty of the sister to call her nurse's attention to
the fact, and help her to attain a truer perception of
the relative claims of her "self" and her "work".
It is far easier for a sister to give in to a request that
she knows to be unreasonable, and which can only be
granted at the expense of throwing additional labour
upon some one else, than to risk a display of temper,
which is not unlikely to follow a refusal. But after
all, a sister must remember that it is not a question
of what is easiest for herself, but of what is best for
her work and really fairest to her subordinate. Whilst
the nurse should be assured that the sister is always
glad to give her pleasure, it would be no true kindness for the sister to allow her nurse to become
selfish, but rather an unconscientious shrinking from

the discharge of an unpleasant duty on the part of
the sister. In the greatly modified conditions under
which hospital nurses are now required to perform
their duties, it would sometimes be hard to discover
where the enormous self-sacrifice of which we *hear*
so much and (sometimes, I fear it must be admitted)
see so little, comes in. Let us avoid by all means
sacrifice for the sake of sacrifice, but do not let us
shrink from sacrifice for love's sake—sacrifice for the
true " love of the work " of which some would-be
nurses are apt to say so much and to show in practice
so little ! The sister must be unselfish on her part
and not hurriedly refuse a special request merely to
avoid the trouble of making some arrangement that
granting it or asking for it to be granted, may involve;
but I am afraid it must be owned that the modern
nurse has a growing tendency to expect that the fair
requirements of the work shall be constantly altered
and adapted to meet her personal wishes, and no good
can result to work or workers from encouraging this
unworthy and unpractical view.   There is always
definite work waiting to be done, and while staff
nurses may fairly claim, and must be encouraged to
take, the regular recreation allotted in their respective
time-tables, any extra recreation is chiefly dependent
upon the sister's wishes and the rules of the institution to which they belong.

My impression is that the temptation to selfishness
in a staff nurse's work does not lie, as a rule, in the
neglect of a patient's wants for considerations of
personal comfort, but this temptation is felt, and, I

am afraid, more or less yielded to almost universally, in the direction of putting off the hardest and least attractive portions of the work upon probationers. In saying this I should be loath to do an injustice to any individual staff nurse who may have earnestly endeavoured to be truly unselfish and conscientious in this respect, but when the question is brought plainly before them, I fear that nearly all must plead guilty to some habitual selfishness in this matter. This is most unworthy of their position and of the high standard of duty that each should at least be striving to attain. The sisters in whose wards this inconsiderate treatment of probationers is permitted are, in my judgment, very gravely to blame. That in some cases they are not aware of the extent to which this petty tyranny is exercised, I can easily believe; but that is the feeblest excuse that can well be brought forward. Ignorance, when it is a plain duty to have knowledge of a subject, can scarcely be regarded as an extenuating circumstance. But if this deplorable system only existed in wards where the sisters could honestly profess ignorance of it, it would be comparatively easy to eradicate it. Unfortunately this is not the case. The strength of this erroneous method of dealing with the relationship of staff nurses and probationers lies in the fact that many sisters openly or tacitly approve of it, candidly stating that a process of merciless " snubbing is good for probationers " ! They are calmly oblivious of how they themselves suffered when going through a similar process, and endeavour to persuade themselves that they are the better for it, forgetting how superfluous they then felt and knew much of it to be.

I shall speak in the next chapter of what I believe to be the best manner of training probationers, and of some of the fallacies prevalent respecting this, but as in practice the work and happiness of probationers is of necessity much influenced by the staff nurses with whom they are so closely associated in their work, it is a matter of considerable importance that the sister should have a clear view of what a staff nurse's duties are towards the probationers. She should endeavour to impress this view upon the former in order to enlist their cordial co-operation, and she must recognise at the same time that it is part of her duty as sister to regulate the treatment which probationers receive at their hands, and to fully acquaint herself with the character and amount of the duties assigned to them. Nothing will produce a thorough and much-needed reform but a just view of the matter on the part of the sister, and a determination to enforce it. She will see at once that the only way to do this effectually is to win the staff nurses to the same opinion, or rather to point out to them that they have lost sight of the nobler possibilities of their work and position, in a selfish misinterpretation of both.

It must become clear to the sister, and be made plain to her nurses, that whatever their personal experiences may have been, that is no reason for perpetuating a bad system. To argue that the treatment of probationers by staff nurses is more or less universally complained of at all hospitals, that the variation between the custom at each one in this respect is rather that of degree than of any fundamental difference, and to add, moreover, what may be said with painful truth, that the moment a probationer is put on staff nurse's duty she follows the example of her fellow-workers, and immediately becomes peremptory with those who are working under her, is merely to prove that a change in the *spirit* which regulates all this is urgently required.

It does not much concern us to inquire how this state of affairs came about. It would appear to have originated partially in the fact that when educated women first entered hospitals they were not cordially received by those already in possession, and it was but natural that nothing should be done to soften difficulties for those who were regarded as unwelcome intruders. Then we may partially account for it by the tendency, inherent in human nature, to exercise all unaccustomed and limited authority somewhat ungently. It needs some strength of character to resist the traditions that we inherit in taking up an office, especially if by so doing we bring upon ourselves an increase of daily work, which otherwise we might inflict upon others, and that, not as an ungracious act of our own, but as a mere matter of custom.

Promotion, in hospital work at any rate, should not be looked upon as an opportunity for laziness, for sparing oneself such duties as may be distasteful, for inflicting upon others treatment that we are

6

eager to escape ourselves, but rather as a means for increased usefulness, for helping and encouraging others, for accepting, as it were, the difficulties that would be overwhelming to new-comers and meeting them ourselves. One of the privileges that promotion confers is the power for rendering greater service. "He that is *greatest* among you shall be your servant." That wise and comprehensive saying will serve as the best illustration of the spirit in which all degrees of promotion should be accepted, and as a true guide for the right line of action when a doubt arises. Hospital nurses can best judge for themselves how far they are inclined to regard their respective duties in this light, and many will quickly learn to adapt themselves to the principle here indicated, not because it is easy—for it is far from that —but because it is right.

If the idea of harmonious working as a family be adopted in the ward, it is manifest directly that the hardest share of the work would not be allowed to rest on the youngest members. Those who are more experienced would think for and spare them, taking some portion of the roughest share of the work themselves. There is no fear that the sort of consideration I mean will spoil probationers, for as soon as they have learnt enough to be put on staff nurses' duty, the same self-denial and thought for others is demanded from them in their turn. It is not fair or reasonable to expect the heaviest burdens to be borne by those who have not yet learned how to lift them, and who are therefore tempted to take an exaggerated view of their weight. Let them grow up sufficiently to grapple with the task awaiting them. But, if the present generation of staff nurses, who should in every way be an example to those now training to come after them, set such a low standard before their eyes, can we wonder that the majority of unthinking workers will follow in their steps, and all that is most deplorable be indefinitely prolonged? So grave a misconception of the treatment best for probationers can but be harmful in its effect upon those who may seek training in the future, or who may be deterred from ever making the attempt, by a dread of what *should* be the *unnecessary* trials that they would have to face.

"Probationers must take their share of rough work," some staff nurses will eagerly and emphatically exclaim. "Certainly they must, but *their* share does not mean your share also and include all the rough work," as most staff nurses appear to think. It will be time for them to take the greater portion when they themselves have become staff nurses, and they will expect to do so, if that is the system upon which they have been brought up. This division of labour is absolutely fair, for it is done by all alike in turn, but in the one case it weighs heavily upon those who are new and inexperienced, and in the other it is carried by those who have become capable of bearing it. I would have every staff nurse make a distinct mental effort to treat all the probationers with whom she comes into personal contact, not as she *was*, but as she *would like to*

have been treated, when she was in that stage of her
hospital existence. If she can manage to retain a
vivid recollection of her own experience, she will
find that her sympathies with new workers become
much enlarged. If this were more generally the
case, should we ever hear of staff nurses sitting
down exclusively together for the sort of second
breakfast or early luncheon which after the 6·30 A.M.
breakfast nearly all hospital workers are glad to get
for themselves? Yet there are staff nurses who do
this, when the morning work is sufficiently advanced,
leaving *probationers* to go on with their work and
get their cup of tea, coffee, or whatever it may be,
when they can, or not at all. On what grounds can
such thoughtless selfishness be justified? Probationers, not being used to the early breakfast,
can scarcely be supposed to need the usual refresh-
ment less; and being unaccustomed to the work,
it is hardly to be imagined that they will find it
less fatiguing than the staff nurses, more particularly if the larger share of it has been left to them.
Again, new probationers are much too shy and
strange, for the most part, to think about making
tea, etc., for themselves, unless they are told to do
so as well as given the opportunity, and naturally a
staff nurse would have no hesitation in getting anything she wanted. By all means let staff nurses
and probationers have their little lunch with such
comfort as circumstances may permit, but let there
be no petty distinctions of this kind, or, if any must
exist, let the positions be reversed, and let the staff

nurses feel that it is their duty to see after the probationers in the first place and themselves in the second.

I might quote other daily incidents of a similar nature, but it is not necessary to go into further details, as this will suffice to show, practically, what a difference I desire to see in the relationship of staff nurses and probationers, and will, I think, give striking proof of the need for a change to take place.

Sisters are ultimately responsible for the training of probationers; but in this, as in other matters in large wards, they are obliged to depend greatly upon staff nurses for help. I would have them both co-operate in the teaching and in the endeavour to show kindness of manner and consideration towards those who, while they are new to the work, find trials in details that others have become indifferent to from familiarity with them. There is no part of a staff nurse's duty to which a sister need pay more attention than her treatment of probationers. The tendency to regard them as necessary evils must be systematically discouraged, and a sister must watch over and prevent the selfishness in this direction which is manifestly such a strong temptation in a staff nurse's work.

I know there is much to be said on the other side of the question, but I reserve that for a later chapter. I will only urge here the importance of a right-minded sister inspiring her staff nurse with a desire to do full justice to every probationer who is placed under her, and express a hope that sisters and staff nurses

will endeavour to remember that all they respectively
do in preparing others to follow in their own footsteps
has a vital influence on the immediate future of the
work to which they, themselves, have thought well to
devote at least some portion of their lives. If a sister
is worthy of her name, she will earnestly watch over
the staff nurses entrusted to her, and let no effort
on her part be wanting to guard against the deterioration which too often takes place in their work and
character, when no special interest is shown in their
individual welfare. I fear most of us can recall instances of nurses who gave promise of better things,
sinking down into the mere routine performance of
their duties, when they have once passed their final
examination and gained their certificate, as though
no further development could be expected and there
were "no more worlds to conquer!" When this
takes place, can we hold the sister wholly blameless?
Why do many staff nurses who have been satisfactory
as probationers, speedily become unpunctual, negli-
gent of minor rules, less eager to offer willing service
to those about them, than when they were probationers, or than many a probationer working under
them, whom it is their plain duty to influence by a
good example in all these details? It would be well
for each sister who can furnish instances of this kind
from her own experience, to reflect on these facts, and
not rest satisfied until she has taken steps to prevent
their recurrence where her influence extends.

There have been occasions when I have been dis-
tressed to perceive how little real interest a sister has

taken in the prospects of a staff nurse who has served under her perhaps for a year, and whom she says she will be sorry to lose. Far from entering sympathetically into the hopes and fears which are naturally involved in the next move of a fellow-worker with whom the sister has been closely associated in daily life, I have known her half surprised that the nurse in question should seek any advice at her hands as to her future plans, and, indeed, if the sister's influence has been so negative throughout, perhaps it *is* rather remarkable that any appeal of the kind should ever have been made!

On these rare occasions, the impression left on my mind has been—not that the sister has meant to be unkind—but that she has wasted invaluable opportunities. Some staff nurses are irresponsive, of course, but there are few indeed who have long resisted or who have ever desired to resist the helpful interest of the sister in their individual work, wishes and prospects. This relationship in work cannot and should never attempt to be forced, but where it exists, it is of infinite service. There must be something seriously lacking in the sister who exercises nothing but this negative sort of influence over any of her subordinates. Sisters capable of taking an active interest in the progress and happiness of those with whom they are working would do well to remember that this kindly personal influence is one of the greatest advantages they can bestow upon those serving under them. In these days there is plenty of easy-going good-nature between the sister of a ward and her staff nurses which sometimes veils the mutual indifference to higher and deeper things, though it is all very well *as far as it goes.*   But it will occur to us all that the mutual interest cannot go very far below the surface if we may infer by the fruits, and it is scarcely unreasonable for earnest workers to ask if that is *all* their sister has to offer them, if that is the *best* they have a right to look for at her hands.

CHAPTER IV.

THE PRACTICAL TRAINING OF NEW PROBATIONERS.

THERE is a great variety in the teaching power of many good sisters, and the art of imparting knowledge with facility is a specially useful qualification for any one desirous of filling these posts. It is impossible that all should be equally successful in this branch of their work, but the first step towards ensuring a better result is to recognise the importance of this duty. There are sisters who permit themselves to speak and think of probationers as though they were their natural enemies. They are not only unreasonable enough to feel aggrieved that they should have the trouble of teaching them, although fully aware on their appointment as sisters that this is one of their most important duties, but they take no pains to conceal this unkindly disposition, and thereby considerably add to the inevitable difficulties that greet every new-comer in her first ward, or when she first goes to any ward in which she has not previously worked. In the latter case the trouble is modified, for if she is not wholly ignorant of hospital doings she may be a shade less unwelcome. Trained nurses, who entertain views of this sort, should never aspire to be sisters, as they are in a

great measure disqualified for the post. The nursing
of patients is the first consideration, they may say,
and so it undoubtedly is, but, if that is the only
portion of their duty that is attractive to them, they
should remain as staff nurses, or seek for a sister's
place in a small hospital where the work is about
equivalent to that of a staff nurse in a large institution. If a knowledge of nursing came by instinct,
there would be no need of sisters as teachers. Wards
could be well managed by staff nurses only, as the
carrying out of the doctor's orders and the general
welfare of the patients might be efficiently ensured
by them. But we know that the thorough technical
training of nurses must be given and acquired in the
wards of a hospital, and that this is a very important
part of a sister's work. That many sisters have felt
this and do feel it there is abundant testimony, both
in the gratitude experienced by many who are now
sisters towards those who have taught them in the
past, and that frequently expressed by probationers,
who are conscious of what they owe towards such
sisters as are taking pains to instruct them in the
present. That it becomes a strain upon the sister's
energy and patience, to be repeatedly imparting the
same items of knowledge to successive numbers of
probationers, is a fact that no one wishes to deny,
and the truth of which will be most felt by those
who are the most unwearied in their exertions.
There is the same kind of temptation to a sister to
refrain from taking the trouble to teach probationers
that are only temporarily working under her, as a

staff nurse finds in the inclination to depute them to do an unfair share of the rougher part of the work, and in both cases the temptation can hardly be too strenuously resisted.

A wider view of the needs of nursing work as a whole, and of their own individual responsibilities in connection with it, would tend to produce more patient perseverance in this matter. Many sisters begin with a desire to teach their probationers well, and are under the impression that they like doing so, but it is disappointing to find how often their interest diminishes when the novelty has worn off. They are apt to forget that the necessity for training probationers is just as great as when they were conscious of it, and were inclined to respond to the call for help which constantly appeals to all who fill a sister's position. It is inevitable that sisters will become comparatively careless and indifferent unless they keep themselves alive to the constant demand for good training which exists. When they realise this they are generally prepared to do their best, for in everything the first step towards supplying a need is to have it distinctly felt. Fortunately few of us are inclined to stand aside and say, "This is no business of mine," if our sympathies have once been enlisted, and if we are assured that, in some measure, we can be of use.

If the question were put plainly to us we should be ashamed not to do our best to forward any cause that we recognised to be good, because our exertions were not likely to bring us any personal credit. Not that this is an element that need be altogether left out of consideration, for as the work is done individually, so the credit eventually comes from and to individuals in many cases, but that is not the most inspiring motive from which to work. To strive eagerly to forward the good of the whole, by unwearied individual exertions, is the duty that each sister should accept. Distinguished physicians and surgeons spare their valuable time and bestow kindly thought and attention on giving that instruction to fresh sets of probationers year after year, which goes so far to qualify them for their work; surely it is for sisters, who have received the benefit of this careful teaching, to supplement in their turn the efforts that are thus patiently made, and to do all in their power to further the same object.

This object is to secure a highly efficient nursing staff for our own hospital in the first place. That implies having a considerable reserve of skilled workers ready to meet the many changes that must inevitably be of frequent occurrence among such a large number. Then we must do our share towards meeting the ever-increasing demand of the public for nursing in all its branches, including the smaller hospitals that have no facilities for training their own workers to succeed others when changes occur. We are distinctly called upon to do our part in a work of considerable magnitude, as we can but acknowledge if we reflect upon the many directions in which it extends. I am anxious that all London Hospital sisters should realise that each one of them has some part in forwarding or hindering it.

But having arrived at a clear perception of this duty, the next step is to discover the best method for its practical achievement, that which will ensure good results to the probationers, which will provide most effectually that none of them shall be neglected, and which will accomplish this with the least trouble to all concerned. The views and practice of the sister as to this matter will be reflected by her staff nurses, we may be sure, and there is no item of the work in which their cordial co-operation is more to be desired.

It is not easy to keep one's sympathies sufficiently awake to be able to put oneself in the place of every new-comer, and to realise even in a remote degree what first impressions are to them. It is manifestly desirable to be able to do this, but if this is more than can reasonably be expected, it is not difficult, and indeed it may be considered absolutely essential, to cultivate the *habit* of giving each fresh worker a kindly welcome. However much this may become a matter of form to the sister, each individual who receives it will be grateful for it; and those who are very shy and retiring will feel an appreciation out of all proportion to the insignificance of the act.

It is not difficult to conceive the state of mind common to many a new probationer on her arrival at the hospital, apart from her individual character. She has probably been kindly welcomed and par-

taken of the usual cup of tea to begin with. She
has been allowed time to unpack, and then finds
herself ready to be taken to the appointed ward.
She wears her uniform for the first time, and
that, being as yet unaccustomed, gives her rather
an awkward, uncomfortable feeling. She is con-
ducted through a building the size of which, while
it is yet strange, appears somewhat bewildering,
and in all probability she is secretly wondering how
she will ever manage to learn her way about it.
If when she is introduced to "sister" she has a
chilling and indifferent reception, the feeling of
desolation that will creep over her is a sensation
that she may smile at afterwards, when she is quite
at home, but one that she will not easily forget, and
that she would not willingly experience a second
time.   Of course the effect will be the same on
the probationer whether the apparent coldness on
sister's part arises because she is engaged with the
doctors, or busy with a bad case, or whether it is
simply a result of the selfish indifference which is
occasionally to be met with, and so much to be
deplored.   But if it is the sister's *habit* to welcome
all new-comers, she will have impressed her nurses
with the importance of kindly greetings, and one of
them will come forward to receive the stranger on
her behalf.   The sister cannot possibly arrange to
be disengaged when probationers arrive, but a little
care in organising what she wishes to be done, by
those who are there to help her when she is not
free, would ensure that no stranger would be left to

feel miserably out of place, with a dozen patients, perhaps, staring at her with the languid curiosity that " a new nurse " is apt to create in their minds, while the " new nurse " herself is feeling awkward and lonely to a degree that varies with her individual character. If the family feeling prevailed, the staff nurses would regard it as simply essential for them to give a kindly reception to all who come to the wards, when the sister is not there, or not at liberty to receive them, as the younger members of a household would do in the absence of the head. Nothing but precept and example on the sister's part will ensure this unfailing courtesy, and the need for it is very great.

Whenever possible it is most convenient and pleasanter for a new probationer to make her first appearance in the wards in or towards the evening. The active press of the work is over, however much in some cases may remain to be done ; and the busy workers can better spare time to say a few words to the new-comer. Moreover, the wards are looking more attractive than they will do at 7 A.M. the following day, when the stranger's introduction to the prosaic side of hospital work begins in unmistakable earnest. Before the new probationer leaves the wards that night the sister should place her under the immediate charge of one of the staff nurses, so that the former may feel that there is some one she may readily appeal to for information respecting the routine of the place. In any case one of the regular workers should take her under her temporary guidance, and do what lies in her power to diminish the loneliness that is inevitably felt to some extent, even under the most favourable circumstances.

It is a possibility for all the nurses and probationers from one set of wards to go off to supper at the appointed hour, leaving a new-comer alone in the wards in all the awkwardness of not knowing whether she ought to go or stay, and certainly not knowing where to go if the former is expected of her! This is an incident which surely reveals an indifference to the amenities of life, and a selfish absorption in one's own concerns to the exclusion of others, to which every woman, who has worked long enough in the hospital to feel at home there, should be ashamed to plead guilty. I do not lose sight of the fact that many strangers may be individually unattractive, and that some who have been at the hospital for a length of time may, notwithstanding, feel a diffidence in speaking to strangers. Still neither of these considerations alters the main fact that some courtesy and kindness is due *to* each one on arrival *because they are strangers*, and that it is due *from* each one who may be brought in contact with them, not so much from personal reasons, as because *they* are in a position to offer it. A double service can be rendered by a kindly suggestion to the stranger that somebody should take her over to supper, for the observation that would naturally come from her guide, "We are not allowed to speak in the passage-wards and corridors," would be an excellent method of impressing this rule upon her from the first, instead of leaving her to find out this and everything else by experience. In saying this I am taking it for granted that they, *whose business it is* to act as guides, are prepared to set a good example in this and other respects, for my suggestions are only offered to those who are sincerely desirous of helping *all* with whom they are brought in contact, by every means in their power.

To the fresh probationer the mere fact of sitting down to supper as one of over a hundred, and of being surrounded by so many strange faces, is a new and not necessarily a pleasing experience, and though the novelty of this proceeding speedily wears off, we may remember that it has to be gone through for the first time by every person who joins the nursing staff. The inquiry whether the new-comer knows how to get to her room, and, perhaps, a kindly promise of calling on the way down to breakfast to bring her there, and to see her safely back to her appointed ward,—the very name of which as well as how to get to it is perhaps a source of perplexity to the stranger,—are merely illustrations of some of the many " little deeds of kindness " that will be acceptable in every case, and often received with disproportionate gratitude for the small effort involved in overcoming natural shyness. There are some to whom these kindly thoughts and expressions come as intuitively as their sympathetic perception of a stranger's needs, but these are comparatively exceptional natures; and I am anxious that each sister

7

should try to inculcate, in some degree, as a duty
upon all her subordinates, unselfish attention to
strangers. Most people may be described as fairly
good-natured and ready to respond to any claim
upon them which does not involve a great deal of
personal trouble, *provided they perceive it,* but it is
useless to expect that the majority of the nursing
staff will think of these things unless their attention is called to them by the sister. Sometimes
her suggestions will be met with the well-known
objection under which a lack of common courtesy
is frequently veiled in hospital life, " I don't like
making friends with new-comers until I know something about them," a very reasonable and commendable precaution, where the shades of character are of
necessity so varied, and where it is almost inevitable
that some, who have been admitted on trial, will not
prove satisfactory. The mistake lies, not in refrain-
ing from an injudicious and probably fruitless attempt
to strike up sudden friendships, but in the failure to
perceive that the fact of being engaged in the same
work under the same roof constitutes a sufficient
reason for mutual acquaintance. The first advance
is due from those who are to some extent at home in
such a great public building as the London Hospital.
The strangeness of the place and ignorance of the
general routine, added to the loneliness which every
new-comer must feel for the first few days, demands
some expression of kindly courtesy during this period
even more than at other times. If a sister thoroughly
realises this herself, she will in time succeed in

making her nurses recognise the importance of it, though in some cases they will be only too slow to do this. She can finally rely upon the indirect help towards establishing this custom which arises from the shame that most people feel, in withholding a kindness that they are conscious is expected of them. The sister will have gained much when she has secured that in her own set of wards, at any rate, the prevailing tendency to selfish indifference is checked by the conviction that better things are looked for from all her workers.

But I am far from meaning to imply that a sister's duty towards probationers is simply to place them under the charge of one of the staff nurses ; that is merely an incident that should not be overlooked in the first instance. To leave probationers entirely to subordinates is a failing that many sisters are only too apt to fall into, and one which should scrupulously be guarded against. It saves the sister trouble, and, it is true, that in many of the details which probationers require to be taught in the first instance, the staff nurses can give the necessary instruction as well as the sister, even if she had time to spare for it. A good sister is only anxious to save herself trouble by such means as may be possible without detriment to her work, not by any system which involves that.

In large hospitals the fact of a probationer being accepted for training, after she has once been received for the usual month's trial, depends in a great measure upon the report of her capabilities and probable suitability for the work which the sister is able to give. It is true that the responsibility of final decision does not rest solely with the sister, but it is essential for those who are anxious to combine the good of the hospital with justice to the individual in question that the head of the nursing department should be able to obtain a definite and reliable opinion from the person who has, or who should have, the best opportunity of judging. The sister should take the utmost pains to prove absolutely trustworthy and efficient in this important matter. Keeping this fact in view would alone make it a clear duty for the sister to see as much of a new probationer as she possibly can, with a view to ascertaining "what she is like," as we familiarly express it.

The point that we are most anxious to be sure of is not whether she knows anything, which is comparatively immaterial at this early stage of her hospital existence, but whether she is capable of learning and eager to do so. The head of the nursing department is obliged to take her knowledge of probationers, and of new workers especially, second-hand, so to speak, as the nature of their respective duties brings them very little into personal contact with her. She may have a distinct impression of what the general characteristics of any selected candidate are likely to be, but she cannot actually know what they are until the facts are elicited by practical experience and laid before her. If a sister realises this, she will understand how necessary it is for her to reproduce as faithfully as possible the impression that any probationer has made upon her own mind. The time and opportunity are hardly sufficient for an infallible conclusion to be arrived at, but it is not too much to ask that each sister shall act to the best of her ability and give this matter her most careful attention. Otherwise she further complicates the difficulty of ascertaining the truth, by handing over the probationer entirely to a staff nurse, so that the opinion given is not even in some measure what the sister thinks from her own observation, but solely what she has gathered from this source, making it third-hand, as it were, when it reaches the head. That the staff nurse should form an opinion and express it freely to sister is only natural and desirable. It would be unwise of the sister not to make use of this means of knowing what the probationer's powers are, but it is still more unwise to be wholly guided by it. I have repeatedly observed in those sisters who, either from selfishness, indifference, or sheer mismanagement, are too much given to adopt this reprehensible plan, how prone they are to quote one of their staff nurse's opinion with blind confidence in its wisdom. They would sometimes appear to absolve themselves by this means from the necessity of exercising their own judgment in the matter, as if it were possible to shirk any of the responsibilities attached to an office, and hold oneself blameless! I have also noticed—what perhaps follows as a matter of course—that such sisters fail to perceive how much the staff nurse's opinion is influenced by the fact of what the probationer knows in the present, or, as the nurse expresses it, "how much use she is," to the exclusion of the real point in question, *i.e.*, what capacity she appears to possess for *becoming of use*. Measured by this unfair standard, a probationer used to house-work, for instance, and ready to take this off the nurse's hands, would be spoken of to sister as a "most promising probationer," though she may be rough, noisy, unperceptive, and lack every other qualification for nursing work, whereas a person who is the reverse of all this, but unaccustomed to house-work, and sadly struggling with the unexpected difficulties which it presents, gets spoken of as "no good at all," and in this way grave, if not intentional, injustice may very easily be done. This is one of the many evils incidental to the fatal habit of allowing the power which rightly belongs to the sister to be delegated to the nurses. Let them take their share —and a considerable one it is where the size of the wards makes the sister busy in other directions—in the training of the probationers, and in finding out what sort of material they are made of, but let them and sister both recognise that the nursing education of the probationers is pre-eminently sisters' work. Moreover, if the staff nurses are as devoted to the sister as is frequently the case, and as the kind consideration they should receive at her hands will go far to ensure, the fact that they are distinctly helping *her*, will go far to induce them to show and to teach probationers all they can.

The health of the probationers—as indeed that of all her subordinates—must be carefully watched

over by the sister, and this is a portion of her responsibilities which she must never lose sight of. I
speak of this more especially as it relates to probationers, because experienced hospital workers will
have grown accustomed to speaking to their sister
when they do not feel well, and will probably be
more alive to the duty of taking care of their own
health. Still a kind, "motherly" sister will see after
all her ward "family" in this respect, and never fail
to report the fact of any of her workers looking over-
tired or needing medical advice.

There is a marked difference in the manner in
which probationers regard their own ailments, as
might be expected from the various characters
amongst them. Some few give in for the "slightest
thing," as we are familiarly told, whereas the difficulty with others consists in their persistent denial
that they are ill, or out of sorts, when this is evidently
the case.

It is better to be truthful and to exercise some
common-sense than to indulge in the imaginary
virtue of "keeping up" when circumstances do not
demand this undue strain. In all probability, it
merely results in the probationer being incapacitated
for duty longer than would have been necessary if
she had spoken out in the first instance, and allowed
those, duly qualified, to judge what was best for her.

This health question—apart from cases of serious
illness—is not quite so simple to deal with as it
may at first appear, and many well-meaning workers
have to learn wisdom in this respect, by their

own personal experience. There are many headaches and minor ailments that those subject to them know will speedily pass off leaving them none the worse, but unfortunately nurses cannot claim immunity from " all the ills that flesh is heir to," and to work on in a condition that they know renders them physically unfitted for the duties required of them, is no true denial of self, but rather an act of senti-mental folly.

Health is one of the essential qualifications for nursing. If a sister kept this view before her pro-bationers, the best of them would perceive the duty of taking reasonable care of their health for the sake of their chosen work. More self-denial may be involved in going out daily in order to keep well, than in keeping up a few hours longer than is necessary with a bad cold or sore throat. It is not intelligent for a healthy probationer, coming, perhaps, from a country home, where she has been accustomed to a daily walk in all weathers, to suddenly relinquish this habit, because she is spending the greater part of her time in wards full of sick people. At the London Hospital we do not accept probationers for regular training until they are twenty-five years of age. Is it too much to expect that when they come to us to learn nursing they should bring with them some common-sense concerning the general management of their own health ? Experienced nurses can recall circumstances where the need for their services has been so great that they have been compelled to tax their own health and strength unduly for a time, but this does not happen in well-regulated hospitals, nor apply to probationers. It is disappointing to an eager worker, interested in her duties, to find herself on the sick list, and often inconvenient to all immediately concerned, but each probationer should grow to feel that we are interested in her individual welfare as well as in her work, and that those temporarily unfitted to nurse others are gladly cared for in their own "home," whilst no one supposes they "wished to be ill" if it could have been avoided.

It is hard on a really kind sister to find that a nurse or probationer whom she was perfectly ready to help has not given her the opportunity when the need existed. Perhaps this would never happen if it were universally understood that this kind of voluntary "martyrdom" is not admired. I am quite ready to believe that this error is well meant, but it is mistaken, and experience proves that the devotion to duty and self-sacrifice implied, is more apparent than real.

A sister must hold herself responsible for the personal neatness of the probationers, as indeed of all working in the wards, from herself to the ward-maids. Sisters would naturally be among the first to criticise the uniform and appearance of the workers in any other institution they may chance to visit, and it is incumbent upon each of them to do all in their power to produce a good result in this respect in the hospital to which they belong. Example and precept must both be employed for this purpose, as both are necessary to secure it. Strict uniform, correctly put on, and great care that cap, apron, and sleeves are as spotlessly clean as circumstances permit, must be enforced. The sister's own habit in these respects will produce its distinct influence when she has occasion to call attention to any defects in the condition of the uniform of her subordinates. If her own appearance is dirty and untidy, it increases the difficulty of reproving others for similar failings. Even if she is not conscious that this is the case, it is inevitable that her reprimands on the subject will not have much weight, while it is probable that they will give rise to reflections unflattering to herself. The object of uniform is not to prevent the wearers looking well, but rather to secure it, and to produce at the same time evidence of that sense of the fitness of things which should characterise dress on all occasions. There is no merit in carelessness about these details, as some persons, curiously enough, appear to imagine. If sisters wear high-heeled, noisy boots and rattling chatelaines, how can they consistently expect their nurses and probationers to refrain from these obviously un-nurselike details ? Many will say that these are mere trifles ; and, in comparison with some other matters, so they are. But I have yet to learn that those other matters are in any way forwarded by the neglect of these comparative trifles, and I am inclined to think that their importance in connection with the work as a whole is apt to be *under*-rather than *over*-rated. They are of distinct value as indications of character, and in the impressions which they give in the many instances in which

externals are the only available means to judge by
at first.

The personal care and general supervision that
apply to other matters will usually ensure the desired
result in the regular workers in the ward, and an
occasional reminder, either in the form of fault-finding,
or of commendation for a neat and business-like
appearance, is all that will be necessary to maintain
it, but the sister must expect a little more trouble in
the case of new probationers. In the first place, they
often do not know what is customary and desirable
in matters connected with personal appearance in the
wards of a hospital, and in the second place, having
no knowledge or experience on the subject, they are
not always willing to be told. There is much in the
manner of telling to soothe or to irritate the possibly
injured feelings of a new probationer, when she learns
that some favourite custom, or item of attire, must
be relinquished, or some other adopted, in conformity
with hospital regulations. Sisters should endeavour
to suggest these things as gently and pleasantly as
possible. In most instances, their wishes will be
readily complied with, but in the rarer cases in
which their suggestions are disputed or resisted,
they must be firm enough to exact obedience. To
insist upon a probationer conforming to rule in the
matter of uniform, has a value in training beyond its
effect upon neatness of appearance. If any small
sacrifice of personal feeling is involved, the readiness
or reluctance with which it is made, will be a revela-
tion of character that an experienced sister will be

quick to note. Those who are not prepared to give up little vanities, or to cheerfully obey in matters of detail, will soon prove to have mistaken their vocation, and must be helped to discover that they have rashly entered upon a career where the denial of " self " is an essential qualification. Some sisters will permit probationers to ignore their duty of adopting the required standard in these matters, not because they approve of their conduct, but from a weak sort of good-natured dislike to speak to them on the subject, or because they have not acquired the art of dealing promptly with such little details. They fail in their duty if they wait for others to complain of what it was for them to observe and remedy. It is a degree more feeble still to say, when inquiries are made as to why such and such things are permitted, that they have spoken to the said probationer on the subject and that she has " taken no notice ". The sister who offers this explanation goes far to pronouncing her own unfitness for the position she fills, when she makes this calm statement of her want of control over her subordinates. In regard to all rules, whether connected with dress or other matters, the sister should make a point of giving kind instruction to the probationer in the first instance not in a fault-finding manner, as though she were to blame for ignorance of what she cannot reasonably be expected to know, but assuming her wish to comply with the regular routine when she understands what it is. I think it is not too much to say that most probationers will respond satisfac-

torily to this line of treatment, but if the sister sees
that her suggestions are not well received, and finds
that they are practically ignored, she must inform
the probationer, when she speaks to her for the
second time on the subject, that if a change does not
take place, it will be the sister's duty to report it as
an act of disobedience.

Many a sister refrains from taking a definite line
of this sort from a well-founded fear of "always
reporting" her probationers, but if the dread of
gaining such an undesirable reputation is well-
founded, the idea that it will arise from this firm
sort of treatment is not. A sister can at once
perceive, if she turns her attention to the matter,
that it weakens her position, or at any rate the
position that she might justly take if she were equal
to it, if she waits to have an obvious failing in one of
her subordinates noticed by others, instead of complaining of it herself. The sister shows herself less
competent than she should be, the fault in the probationer has remained unchecked, and the sister has
finally to speak to her from a less dignified standpoint
than she need have done in the first instance. The
ward in which the sister consistently carries out the
system suggested will not be one where "reporting"
is prevalent, but, on the contrary, one where it rarely
occurs. This may not be the case at first, but it will
be established very shortly, if the sister has the
perseverance and foresight to act decidedly and in
the straightforward, kindly manner that I here
venture to recommend. "What sister says" will

have double weight, if they are sure that she will do
what she says. Her authority will be incalculably
strengthened if she speaks with the conviction in
herself and her hearers that she will be promptly
upheld, as will certainly be the case, when she acts
with this firmness and judgment. Those who are
inclined to be troublesome and argumentative may
prefer to yield at once when they are convinced that
they will be compelled to do so ultimately, and it is
evident that those who are inclined to prolong their
insubordination should not be allowed to do so. It
is desirable for the sake of all concerned, that the
sister should not permit her authority to be set at
defiance, and she may rely upon it that her difficulties
will speedily increase, if she is weak enough to wait
until she herself is found fault with, for a lack of due
control over the subordinates for whose obedience to
rule she is responsible, instead of being the first to
complain if, as should rarely happen, her efforts have
been set at nought.

I have often thought, when I have seen good-
natured but injudicious sisters reluctantly compelled
to report at last, when they should have done so in
the first instance, how much worry and annoyance
they would spare themselves if they were wise
enough to adopt some such system as this. If
they were sufficiently consistent in their dealings
with those working under them, they would all
entertain the wholesome conviction that obedience
to sister was essential, and the consequences of
disobedience, not problematical, but certain. Every

sister who acts on this principle is showing the
truest kindness to those who work under her, as
well as ensuring the best results for the discipline
of her wards.

The sister must take an early opportunity of giving
her probationers such hints in reference to hospital
manners, as experience shows her to be necessary. All
evidence of frivolity must be sternly repressed, as wholly
unsuited to the surroundings and unworthy the wearer
of a nurse's uniform. On the other hand, cheerfulness, contentment, and courtesy must be sedulously
cultivated. She must never scold for pardonable
ignorance on this or any other subject, but she
should remember that it is her business to remove
this ignorance as speedily as possible. If in doing
this she can manage to instil those feelings of
esprit de corps which will sometimes act as an
inspiring motive something definite will have been
gained. Principles of loyalty are eminently con-
tagious, and if a sister is greatly influenced by such
considerations herself, others will gradually be inclined
to accept them as a matter of course. The higher
the motive that can be given and accepted for the
obedience that must inevitably be exacted from the
members of a large community of workers, the
easier the enforced conformity to rule is likely to
prove.

The sister should make a point of seeing as much
as she is able of her probationers, and do all she can
to establish kindly relations with them. Many an
excellent trained nurse or sister can tell how nearly

she was giving up the profession altogether at the beginning, but for the kindness and opportune encouragement of some sister whom she invariably speaks of in terms of the heartiest gratitude. If the object of our lives is to help our fellow-creatures, it is a thousand pities that *any* of the innumerable ways in which a hospital sister can help others should be thrown away, because she fails to perceive how much rests in her hands.

There are sisters who, instead of this sympathy with the inevitable trials of a beginner, act as though their one object was to disgust them with the work they have aspired to excel in, and, although we may endeavour to believe that this is far from their deliberate intention, the effect upon the unlucky probationer is much the same as if it were.

Some few of the best probationers — shall we admit that perhaps they are not a large proportion? — enter the wards with an impression that the sister under whom they are to serve must be a woman who cannot fail to win their deepest respect, if not their cordial admiration and affection ; such a woman as they may humbly hope to become in a distant future when they have been taught the innumerable things they need to learn, and have worked, as they mean to work, with the view of one day deserving the title of a thoroughly trained nurse. When such a disposition exists on the part of a probationer it is favourable to progress if she falls into good hands. What shall we say of the sister who renders it impossible for any intelligent person to retain that view after working in her wards for a day or two? She has more to answer for than she would like to believe.

Considerable allowance should reasonably be made for the gloomy views which a new probationer is apt to take of the prospects before her, on the ground of the depressing effect of the physical fatigue, caused by the unaccustomed labour. The aching feet, that at first grow almost too painful to walk upon in some cases, are the reverse of exhilarating, and although these troubles are transient, they are very real while they last. We are also prone to forget that the first glimpse of the prosaic side of hospital life is likely to be very disenchanting. It is superfluous for us to do anything to darken it further. There is no need to check the previously conceived enthusiasm for it, which, if real, will prove invaluable to the beginner, and the reality of which is about to receive a very practical test. A staff nurse who feels a pride in the condition of her ward may well make light of the trouble of sweeping, and even find a satisfaction in her power of doing this quickly and well, just as a probationer rejoices in having taken "nurse's duty for a half-day" satisfactorily, and cheerfully performs under these circumstances every detail of the work that had thus fallen to her share. But I cannot be surprised or disappointed that a newcomer is not conscious of any rapture at the sight of a broom, nor is even filled with joy at the prospect of learning how to handle it properly! I have no sympathy with the probationer who refuses to do

8

what she is told, or who entertains objections to doing hard or rough work because she imagines that it is "beneath her," or that it "isn't her place," or any other vulgar notion of this sort, but I can readily understand the repugnance that she feels towards many unattractive duties at first, and the difficulty she experiences in getting accustomed to them. That all the knowledge she is acquiring will prove more useful in the future than she has any idea of is more than probable, but it is only in the future that she will derive consolation from that fact, and those who are able to see further should do all they can to look at the hardships from her point of view in the present, whilst guiding her to look beyond it. A staff nurse, in doing the rougher portions of her work, has compensation in the interests of her more strictly nursing duties, and the affection of her patients, not to speak of the credit that is justly hers for the good condition of her ward and everything in it; but it will be remembered that a new probationer has none of these alleviations, and to her the day's work frequently appears unmitigated drudgery. Probationers must begin from the first to take their share in all the work that has to be done, and I have not the slightest desire to prevent this. I would only stipulate that their share should be a considerate one, and ask the sisters to observe in many instances how far this is from being the case unless they take the trouble to ensure it.

I am willing to believe that some sisters have adopted and permitted a comparatively harsh line of treatment towards new probationers from an honest, though, as I think, wholly mistaken conviction, that it was the best course to pursue, but I fail to perceive any advantage to be gained by it. I have given this matter long and very careful consideration, but I have *never* seen any results from this system that I would wish to see emulated by others, and I *have* seen much that I should earnestly desire to be studiously avoided. Those sisters who have occasionally advocated that the hardest methods of dealing with probationers produce the best results in the long run, and have urged, by way of proving this, that they themselves were subjected to similar treatment, have, curiously enough, been striking illustrations of its pernicious effect, and have gone far to strengthen my convictions in the opposite direction, by the practical proof their daily lives have sometimes afforded of what I should *not* wish any probationers or sisters to be or to become. Systematically harsh treatment seldom arises from kindly and unselfish motives, and I would fain abolish everything that originates in less worthy conceptions from the wards of a hospital. " The woman is so hard upon the woman," is an unpalatable side of the truth that we are reluctant to have forced upon us under any circumstances, and least of all amidst those surroundings where hardness and every form of selfishness are conspicuously out of place.

The sister will get much more help of the right kind from her staff nurses for the training of probationers if she makes them feel that it is a matter which claims a good deal of attention from her. The

frequent inquiry from sister that she wonders if such
and such a probationer is learning anything, or
whether she knows how to do such and such things,
would go a long way towards making the staff nurses
feel that it was incumbent upon them to teach her.

Even a new probationer, if she is a month in one
set of wards, should have been taught the rudiments
of the kind of nursing required for the class of
cases allotted to the charge of that sister.   In
medical wards a probationer should learn at least
how to take a temperature, how to make and apply
poultices and fomentations, how to make the bed of
a helpless patient, some methods adopted for the
prevention of bedsores, the correct reading of the
scales of measurement on the various glasses in use
in the wards, and sundry other details of a similar
nature.   There are always opportunities of learning
these simple things, though it may take a longer
period to see, and more knowledge on the part of a
probationer to understand, the special nursing for
different cases, and to feel an interest in the treatment.
No sister in charge of medical wards should be
satisfied to let a new probationer leave her, at the
end of a month, ignorant of any one of the ordinary
routine details that I have mentioned, and of others
that will doubtless suggest themselves to her.

In like manner any probationer who was sent into
a surgical or accident ward should know something
of bandaging in a very short time ; she should also be
taught the names and uses of the commoner surgical
instruments, the manner of preparing dressings, and

the names of many of the applications in general use, while some little information should be given as to the objects for which they are employed. It is almost incredible how long probationers may sometimes be in the wards of a hospital, and remain absolutely ignorant of what each one should be familiar with very shortly after her admission. This may be partly owing to a want of intelligence on the part of the newcomer, but in the majority of cases it is more justly to be attributed to the want of system, and sometimes to the complete absence of anything approaching painstaking instruction on the part of the sister. Every sister in charge of surgical wards should feel herself to blame if a probationer, even one who is quite new to the work, leaves her wards at the expiration of four or five weeks in ignorance of these rudimentary details of surgical nursing. Neither must the sister rest contented with the *probability* that the probationer has learned these and other essential items connected with this branch of her work. She must ascertain beyond question that this is the case. There is much that can only be acquired in the course of experience, and in the light of increased knowledge, but such matters, as those to which I refer, can always be taught, to any one desirous of learning, in connection with the practical nursing of the patients consigned to almost any set of surgical wards. A minute or two of conversation, on what a probationer had probably learnt in their ward when she was leaving it, would prove both an encouragement and reminder to sister and nurse. Everything which tends to bring this subject before them from a practical point of view should be constantly encouraged, as the need for untiring effort on their part is continuous. As a rule probationers are eager to learn, and grateful for being taught, two points distinctly in favour of the teachers, and the exceptions are not worth much consideration.

Sisters and staff nurses are both very apt to forget how utterly strange and incomprehensible to a new-comer are the names of instruments and other terms in common use in a hospital. The most inconsiderate manner, perhaps, in which this fact is frequently illustrated, is by sending the strange probationer on hurried messages for articles of which she does not know the name, the appearance, or, perhaps, even the object for which they are wanted. She arrives at the place where she has been sent to fetch them, in a state of hopeless bewilderment, and the chances are that she is obliged to go back without them, and reluctantly explain that she could not make herself understood. If the doctors are waiting for what she has failed to bring, the inconvenience is general, the sister is naturally irritated by the delay and apparent confusion, and the probationer is vexed and uncomfortable that she should appear so helpless and stupid. Yet, is the stupidity evinced in the proceeding to be fairly ascribed to her? Ignorance and a failure to understand hurried and unfamiliar directions give the appearance of stupidity, but it by no means follows that this is really the case. A little care on the part of those who give the order might spare the probationer a painful experience, and others a perfectly avoidable delay. If staff nurses knew that they would have to do all the errands until probationers were familiar with the names of what is usually required, and of where these articles are to be found, some of them might find this an additional reason for bestowing more instruction upon these points. Probationers should not be sent to fetch they know not what, from they know not where, when the required article is needed without delay, but should learn their way about by accompanying others in the first instance, and then by fetching what may be wanted when there is no immediate hurry for it, and they can go a second time if the right article is not forthcoming on their return to the ward.

But while I think a considerate tone towards the probationers very desirable from every point of view, I have no idea of spoiling them—as some sisters may fear when they have read as far as this—and nothing is further from my wish than that they should lose half the value of their training by laxity of discipline. I have observed with a degree of wonder that such sisters as are least kind to their probationers are also least particular with them in many essential respects, and that they permit irregularities that more amiable sisters would never dream of passing over. This fact can only be accounted for on the supposition that such sisters are altogether more indifferent to the real welfare and advancement of their probationers.

Many new-comers display an indifference to exact punctuality, and to paying careful regard to the wishes of those under whom they are placed, which is surprising to those who have learnt the value of accuracy in such matters. If the sister is impressed with the importance of teaching the duty of perfect obedience to the rules laid down, her views will be speedily reflected in the minds of her probationers, and will produce an effect upon them.

A sister should always inquire from a new probationer if she has read her rules and understands them, or if there is anything in them that she would like explained to her. The mere question would convey to the probationer a fresh sense of their importance, and would probably lead to another perusal of them at the earliest opportunity. Moreover, if the sister insisted that the probationer should take the trouble to read her rules over again, whenever she found that one of them had been transgressed, not only would the few rules that exist become more familiar, but the necessity of honourable obedience to them would be more impressed upon the probationer's mind, and that is the real point to be achieved. If a sister felt this to be a distinct portion of her duty, not only would the general order and discipline be increased satisfactorily, but probationers would escape the more serious trouble, which they sometimes fall into when the breaking and ignoring of rules has become so habitual with them as to attract attention ; and then, perhaps, it becomes impossible to allow the delinquent to remain in the training school, lest the general discipline should suffer thereby.

In short, sisters should endeavour to exercise a beneficial influence over their probationers in *every* part of their hospital life. That some will prove unworthy of the pains expended upon them is a melancholy fact, but one that does not in the least alter the necessity for the sister to do her utmost for the probationers as a whole. That she will reap a rich reward in the efficient work and deep gratitude of many there can be no doubt. Her unselfish efforts to benefit others by her own knowledge and experience will be productive of much good that will encourage her to persevere, and of much of which she may never know, though it will not be of less value to others on that account.

I would urge all sisters to take their probationers on the best side of their nature, appealing to the highest motives which they appear capable of understanding. We none of us want our daily work put before us on lower considerations than those upon which we are naturally inclined to see it. Never attempt to crush out enthusiasm for a work that is ever beautiful, if viewed in connection with the love and self-sacrifice it calls forth in those devoted to its service. Rather strive to enhance this enthusiasm by giving it a practical shape, and proving in your own person that a long or short course of hospital work has had no tendency to dull sympathy, or engender any want of what we understand by the term "womanliness," but that it has only tended to deepen those qualities in human nature which rightly claim our deepest reverence and admiration.

People ignorant of hospital work may and often do indulge in ludicrously romantic notions concerning it, but we who are in the midst of it all, who are spending our days amidst the grave realities of life, death and suffering, need not fear that we shall justly be accused of indulging in too high-flown ideas when we are actually engaged in the practical, prosaic and, as some would say, revolting details of which nursing in a great measure consists. Do not let us turn or attempt to turn others from the noblest way of regarding it. Instead of shrinking from so-called high-flown thoughts, rather let us soar towards them. We shall get the clearest view over the valley if we ourselves are standing on the heights. I would say to every sister in dealing with those who look to her for guidance—

> " *Be* noble, and the nobleness that lies
>   In other men, sleeping but never dead,
>   Will rise in majesty to meet your own ".

CHAPTER V.

THEORETICAL TRAINING OF MORE ADVANCED PROBATIONERS.

LARGE and small training schools for nurses have their respective advantages and disadvantages. In each we must accept the defects of their qualities and do what may be possible to minimise these.

Our large training school offers unrivalled opportunities for wide and varied practical experience, and has other undoubted merits that it is needless to enumerate here. On the other hand, the size of the wards forced upon us by the plan on which the building was erected, necessitates the allotment of a large number of beds (fifty to sixty) to the charge of one sister, and this fact—undesirable in itself—involves many exceptional arrangements.

Sisters with four wards containing some sixty patients under the care of half-a-dozen different physicians or surgeons—according to the nature of the cases for which the set of wards is reserved— can scarcely be regarded as practical head nurses in the ordinary sense of the term. They *are* head nurses of course, and actively responsible for the nursing of every patient in their wards, but with so many patients, nurses and probationers to supervise, a large portion of their daily work consists in seeing

(123)

that all treatment ordered has been efficiently carried out, rather than in directly serving the patients themselves. This does not imply that the sister never does any actual nursing herself. She should always be or endeavour to become the best practical nurse in her wards, but it means in practice that the sister of such large wards has only time to undertake a small share in *doing* what is ordered for the patients, and is obliged to devote herself chiefly to the task of seeing that all of them are well cared for.

In smaller wards (thirty beds) sisters are able to take a larger share in the actual nursing of their patients, which is more in accordance with the generally-accepted view of a head nurse's duties, and always a preferable arrangement when there is any choice in the matter.

The only thing that can be said in favour of the large set of wards is that the charge of them forms an excellent preparation in many respects for some of the duties which fall to a matron's share in smaller hospitals. Many a useful institution throughout the country does not contain more than sixty beds, and the same system of management may to a great extent be applied to hospitals containing double or treble that number, so that experience gained in the capacity of "sister" here may prove of special service to those intending to serve as matrons later on.

This variety in the size of our wards, and the consequent difference in some respects in the duties assigned to those filling the office of sister, enables those in charge of comparatively small wards to take

a larger share in the theoretical training of probationers, while those sisters with large wards under
their care have greater opportunities for imparting
practical instruction to probationers during the performance of their ward and nursing duties.

When probationers become sufficiently advanced to
be put on "special" duty, *i.e.*, in charge of some important case under the supervision of the staff nurse
and sister, great pains must be taken to teach them
how to keep a clear business-like record of their case,
and how to report fully and concisely all that is to
be known concerning it. Every capable sister will
utilise these opportunities for ascertaining beyond
all doubt that the probationer has learnt, or is
rapidly learning under active supervision how and
what to observe, and how to record *facts* briefly and
methodically. She must teach her the best and
simplest system of recording the treatment ordered,
the remedies that have been actually applied, or a
distinct statement of when they will be due. All
particulars concerning nourishment, stimulants or
medicine must be so clearly stated that there need
never be the slightest difficulty in having this information ready for the doctor at any moment, nor
in the "nurse," who relieves the other "special"
for night or day duty, understanding exactly *where*
she takes up the case.

The probationer must be required as far as possible
to copy out her "cases" in her own note-book for
careful correction afterwards, and for future reference,
when she has had time to appreciate more fully the

value of careful teaching in this essential part of her training. Progress in " case taking " will be a useful indication to those who feel themselves responsible for the probationer's training, as to how far she is being well taught, how far she is profiting by the opportunities afforded her, and as to what knowledge of nursing she has acquired. The principles on which case taking should be carried out—the best form of recording facts—can be easily taught by the class sister as well as the ward or night sister, but how and what to observe beyond the technical details common to all cases, can only be effectually taught by the sister in charge of the patient in question. Some sisters are simply admirable in the manner in which they impart this knowledge, and in the skilful way in which they either draw out or direct the latent powers of observation in any intelligent pupil, or stimulate an unobservant person to greater effort. All sisters cannot be equally gifted as teachers, but all may learn to recognise that they have a distinct duty in this direction, and endeavour to perform it to the best of their ability.

In small training schools it is comparatively easy for the matron to take an active part in the individual training of the probationers, but where large numbers have to be provided for, she can only, for the most part, give them theoretical instruction collectively, and make such careful arrangements as may be possible for their systematic individual class teaching, by sisters specially selected for the purpose.

It is very desirable that these sisters should perceive the nature and importance of the task allotted to them, and spare no pains to fit themselves for its adequate fulfilment.

What are the qualifications needed for the success of a class sister?

Let me quote the able definition of a skilled writer on this subject :—

"1. That they must know thoroughly what they propose to teach.

"2. That they shall have a strong desire—a desire of the heart—to teach what they know.

"3. That they shall have a living, kindly, and sympathetic interest in the *minds* which they teach.

"4. That in teaching they shall think of those minds first, of their subject second, and of themselves and their own cleverness not at all." [1]

If those sisters who are trusted with the inspiring responsibility of taking classes, would keep these four essential points, so admirably and clearly defined, steadily before them, it would be superfluous to enlarge upon the advantage which could not fail to follow for all concerned. If the fulfilment of these complete and simple directions cannot be expected from all who are required to take classes, at any rate, each sister must refrain from accepting

[1] *Teachers' Guild Addresses, and the Registration of Teachers*, by S. S. Laurie, LL.D., Professor of the Theory, History and Art of Education in the University of Edinburgh.

any lower standard as "good enough". It may safely be said that the degree in which these essential qualifications are possessed will be the measure of the success which will attend each teacher's instructions. At the London Hospital, a class of probationers rarely exceeds six in number, and this limit has been adopted to enable the teaching given to be thoroughly individual in character. A quiet hour with the same six probationers once a week should certainly enable an intelligent sister to form a clear idea of the capabilities and characteristics of each of her pupils before many weeks have elapsed, and the keen interest she must endeavour to feel and to show in the progress of each one will be the best guide as to the exact nature of the help required at her hands.

The lectures which form the ready-made subject, so to speak, of each week's class are delivered on a carefully arranged system, and it is the business of the class sister to see that each probationer is thoroughly well grounded on the system laid down. She must check the very general tendency of her pupils to wander from the matter in hand, to subjects which they may happen to think more interesting, and, generally speaking, she should not anticipate the instructions of the lecturers, but rather, if time permits, go over old ground, if the matter of the last lecture has been effectually disposed of. Every examination proves that this might have been done more frequently with advantage. Nothing but the guidance of an experienced sister can enable a probationer to confine her attention in the first instance to the sort of knowledge that she must acquire, in order to become proficient in her own work. There is always a risk, without this guidance, that an industrious probationer will spend time and energy in desultory study, that will not aid her in the object she has at heart, but rather tend to confuse her mind and memory with scraps of ill-assorted information, that are more likely to mislead and hinder than to help her in her practical duties.

All this the class sister must see to, giving such advice as the degree of progress a probationer has made and her general capabilities may indicate.

The class sister must teach probationers how to write out their lectures fully from the notes they take at the time. She should occasionally give them two or three questions to answer in writing, allowing them to take the answers from books or wherever they like, by way of impressing any special information upon them, and requiring that the papers brought to her are in the exact form of an examination paper. This enables each one to become familiar with such details as writing on one side of the paper only, leaving a margin, putting the number of the question instead of wasting time by copying it, etc., etc., items almost too small to mention, but which have their relative importance when examination days come, and which are not altogether trivial to those probationers who have had less general education than the majority of our workers, but who yet

9

may be able to acquire the knowledge necessary for a trained nurse.

The class sister should insist that all technical terms misspelt are written out several times at the other end of the lecture book, to prevent any repetition of the error.

She should advise each probationer to provide herself with a small rough note-book to carry in her pocket, and encourage her to write in this any question that may occur to her, leaving the opposite page blank for the answer to be inserted later on. This answer may be obtained from the ward sister, the night sister, or the class sister, as opportunity offers, and the answer may occasionally be long delayed, but if the probationers are intelligent, and their teachers patient and energetic, it will ultimately be forthcoming. Such a little volume as this, carefully, however roughly, kept throughout the training of almost any probationer, could scarcely fail to be interesting as well as instructive to the possessor of it. A half-amused glance at it in future years might serve to renew her sympathy with beginners and revive useful memories.

Probationers should also be encouraged to copy the technical names and medical terms they come across in their work, looking up the exact meaning of them at the earliest opportunity. A probationer is far more likely to remember them, and how to spell them correctly, if she writes them down in the first instance, at one end of her little rough note-book, and the fact of having such items written down in her pocket will enable a probationer to renew her acquaintance with them at many an odd minute until they become perfectly familiar to her.

These simple means of speedily acquiring knowledge will frequently be wasted unless the probationer is guided to utilise them *from the very beginning*, and while all sisters share in the responsibility of teaching probationers, the class sister has undoubtedly the best opportunity for definitely ascertaining in the case of each of her pupils that no time is lost in adopting all the means which are likely to prove conducive to progress.

Generally speaking, class sisters find their pupils eager to learn, but it would be a mistake to suppose that this is invariably the case. In these days probationers "take up hospital work" from such varied motives, that it is not remarkable that mutual disappointment should sometimes be the result. Some merely desire to gain a certificate in a given time, and wish to do and to learn as little as possible consistent with achieving that end. Some are indifferent and careless from sheer idleness, and a want of previous training in the habit of devoting themselves heartily to any task that they have undertaken. Some are quick and superficial—contented with a mere surface knowledge and not willing to take the pains necessary to gain the valuable quality of thoroughness. Some are slow but by no means stupid, and atone for the trouble needed in repeating explanations by the way in which they retain knowledge that they have once grasped. On

the other hand, some are hindered by their own
conceit, and meet the sister's patient exhortations
to exert themselves, by vague assurances that they
"really understand everything, only somehow or
other they cannot manage to explain it!" or in reply
to her remonstrances over a badly-written lecture,
they will take refuge in repeated declarations that
their practical work is excellently done, a statement
which is usually found to mean that it is done
entirely to their *own* satisfaction, rather than to the
satisfaction of those better qualified to form an
opinion on the matter.

These, and other types of probationers which
might easily be added by way of illustration, are
familiar to every class sister, as well as the cheerful, earnest worker, whom she at once recognises as
promising material for the making of a trained
nurse. She has to do her best with those of average
ability as well as with the more promising probationers, and should remember how much the final
result of their hospital training will eventually be
due to the influence she is able to obtain over each
one of them. She must be firm and true as well as
kind in her respective dealings with them; indeed
there can be no true kindness shown without these
essential qualities. She must help them to get rid of
such delusions respecting their work, or their own
personal qualifications for it, as she perceives to be
hindering their progress, and she must be simply
unwearied in her endeavours to keep a true view of
the work, and its inherent nobility, steadfastly before

them. A few minutes taken from the technical instruction (which is the main object of the class) would be well spent in pointing out in general terms some true advance in the workers which the sister has observed with pleasure, or some opportunities of serviceable self-denial which her hearers have failed to perceive,—some detail of hospital discipline the object of which is not sufficiently appreciated by those for whose benefit it is designed—time so bestowed in the right spirit will never be wasted, nor can it ever fail to produce *some* of the effects hoped for. Sisters who make the effort required to bring forward these truths, tell me again and again of the encouragement that the ready response they are certain to receive from some, if not all, of the class has been to them, and it has not infrequently happened that those who have appeared the least responsive have not been the last to profit by the opportune assistance. Many excellent sisters find it hard to realise that the hospital life, so familiar to them, is strange and full of perplexities to those just entering upon it, so they forget to put into words, facts and principles that may be guiding their own lives, but which the probationer, however eager and willing, cannot be expected to perceive in the first instance for herself.

To the inexperienced beginner many of her daily duties appear a waste of time, many of the necessary regulations for the orderly working of a large institution appear merely vexatious restrictions, the exact punctuality and personal neatness required, appear

to her irritating, and even nonsensical, if the young
woman in question is not of a very reflective turn of
mind. Such hasty, mistaken views, following the
first plunge into the hospital world, are not incom-
patible with many good and nurse-like qualities in the
background. A wise sister will remember this fact,
and tell her class plainly that she understands the
novices' point of view, and does not expect them to
be able to form a sound judgment upon such
matters. She can explain to them that she expects them to have sufficient common-sense to
cheerfully accept such conditions as have been
laid down for them, by those who *can* speak with
the experience *they* have yet to acquire. She can
turn their attention to the qualities which all women
who aspire to become nurses are required to possess
in a marked degree ; such as self-control, promptitude,
punctuality ; and all those other characteristics which
go to make up the complete reliability, without which
no woman can be really serviceable as a nurse ; and,
she can guide them to see that these essentials have
to be patiently *acquired,* and cannot be complacently
put on with the probationer's new uniform. These
facts are so simple that it might well be thought all
would perceive them for themselves, but experience
teaches us that they need saying, and that a patient
repetition of them is often necessary, if we would
give each new-comer a fair start on the right road.
The opportune utterance of these truths, in some
form or other, is a very literal smoothing of the path
for those setting forth for the first time, and when

the guidance comes from those who have already travelled by the same way, it will for the most part be readily and, indeed, gratefully accepted. After all, probationers are not the only persons who need to be frequently reminded that the indirect means, tending towards the achievement of an object, are often as valuable as those which we can perceive for ourselves are leading us directly towards it.

> " For miracles are ceased ;
> And therefore we must needs admit the means
> *How* things are perfected."

Let sisters keep this fact impressed upon their probationers, and many a distasteful task, or commonplace duty will be gladly performed, as they learn to realise its relative value in fitting them for the end they have in view. Most probationers will admit that it would take nothing short of a miracle, to inspire them instantaneously with those qualities that we love, admire and reverence in a loving woman who has become a perfect nurse !

Those who wish to study other arts appear to have less temptations to instruct their chosen teachers as to the best means of teaching *them* the principles of the art in question, than is sometimes the case with those who wish to learn the art of nursing. Beginners select the training school they wish to enter, leaving no stone unturned to secure the eagerly sought after vacancy. Once admitted, some probationers are loud in their expressions of surprise, that every detail is not arranged in accord-

ance with their preconceived notions. They noisily
exchange their opinions with other probationers—as
new and ignorant as themselves—and descant freely
upon the very different means *they* would adopt of
teaching a subject about which, be it remembered,
the young critics are at this time wholly ignorant!
Would any pupil who desired to become a true artist
in painting or music allow herself to behave in this
unreasonable manner? Scarcely, I think; nor would
many probationers be inclined to do so, if sisters
took the trouble to perceive this not altogether
uncommon tendency, and point out the folly, which
many will quickly recognise as such, if they are
allowed to catch a glimpse of themselves through
more experienced, but ever kindly eyes. Unless
the class sisters themselves have mistaken their
vocation, they will spare no pains to inspire their
probationers with an ardent enthusiasm for their
work, and lead them to see that to become "worthy
of the vocation wherewith they are called," demands
their best endeavours. Many will admit this in
the abstract, but it is for the sisters to bring
the fact home to them, in one practical shape after
another, in the midst of their daily work.

Class sisters, who are constantly setting a high
standard of duty before their probationers, will insensibly be helped thereby to approach more nearly to
their own ideals, and they must remember that
precept is helpful and necessary as well as example
—a fact that too many, whose business it is to teach,
are often apt to forget. The instruction classes

will be eagerly looked forward to by teacher and pupils, if the sister makes these occasions what they ought to be, and establishes the easy relationship which should exist between those who are eager to learn and those who are able and willing to teach. Each class sister at the London Hospital holds two or three classes during the week, so that she may have altogether a dozen or eighteen pupils whom she is preparing for examination. She must herself attend the weekly lecture, take full notes and conscientiously prepare herself, by careful study, for the efficient fulfilment of this branch of her duties. It is needless to add that when the right woman discharges this important task to the best of her ability, her well-deserved reward is not far to seek.

If the sisters in charge of smaller wards have the largest share in grounding the probationers in a thorough knowledge of a trained nurse's duties, it falls to the share of the sisters of the larger wards to give special instruction to those who are further advanced. When an intelligent woman has acquired a sufficient knowledge of her work, and displayed such characteristics as lead those in authority to hope that, with further training and experience, she may develop into a capable hospital sister, she can scarcely have a greater advantage than to be placed as assistant sister in a set of wards managed by a clever, experienced worker, and there must be some strange deficiency in the young sister if she does not profit by her exceptional opportunities, to learn more than she had previously believed possible.

Of course, much will depend upon the teaching power of the ward sister, and her willingness to exercise it on behalf of the new-comer, but the beginner will be gravely to blame if she does not learn a great deal from her own observation, in addition to that which she is directly taught.

It is found that few form any idea of a sister's duties until they put on her uniform, and it is many a long day after that, generally speaking, before anything like an appreciation of the true nature of a sister's responsibilities comes to the unaccustomed worker. I do not mean that the routine duties are not easily and, for the most part, quickly acquired, but an earnest woman placed in this position of trust, and allowed to share responsibilities of which she has hitherto had no adequate conception, is undergoing a most valuable preparation for future work.

We seldom enter very keenly into the difficulties of any office which we have never filled, and, as a rule, the probationer has almost everything to learn about a *sister's* duties, as distinct from the actual nursing of her patients. Her idea of the use of sister, hitherto, has been to go to her in all emergencies, to accept sister's decision as final in all matters appertaining to her ward and patients, and to require every one else to do the same. But when it comes to being appealed to oneself, instead of asking for guidance, when it rests with oneself to give a decision in perplexing circumstances, instead of having clear directions on which to act, it gradually dawns upon the untried sister that responsibility is not an unmixed delight, and that time and careful preparation are both necessary to ensure any success worthy of the name.

A sensible ward sister will get much useful assistance from an " assistant sister," whilst giving her the necessary instruction in ward management. It means that a trained nurse is free and ready to help the sister in her own work, and in our large busy wards such help is generally welcome. Of course tact is necessary on the part of the new-comer, and she must avoid the two extremes of being too forward in taking the sister's place, or of never lending a helping hand unless she is distinctly asked to do so. But tact is an essential qualification for any one aspiring to be a sister, and this is only one of the many directions in which it must be exercised.

The assistant sisters are required to make themselves familiar with every detail of a sister's duty, and they can only do this by rendering practical assistance in the actual performance of these duties ; by carefully observing all that is required from the sister of the ward, and seeking her explanation, as opportunity offers, of anything they fail to understand. Possible contingencies may present themselves to the mind of a beginner, and she must choose her opportunity for discussing them with the sister, and endeavour to gain all she can from her experienced guidance.

The ward sister must take care that assistant sisters pay special attention to the more domestic, as distinct from the strictly nursing side of ward management. They should be required to constantly inspect the condition of the test-tables, lavatories, sculleries, ash-pails, etc. the manner in which the duties of the ward maid are performed, the disposal of the soiled linen, and the condition of linen returned from the laundry, and many other things which it would be superfluous to enumerate. They must be carefully instructed in the clerical work for which a sister is responsible, and, to ensure efficiency in this respect, the ward sister must allow her pupil to fill up the daily papers under her supervision, as far as this can conveniently be done. Routine duties become easy with practice, and it is an immense advantage if a young sister has grown familiar with all such details before she is entrusted with "holiday duty," and makes the next advance in her training for a permanent post of responsibility.

It is not desirable that the assistant sister should use the sister's room, for her constant presence might become a weariness to the ward sister, whom she should always endeavour to help by every means in her power, in return for the trouble which her special instruction in one sense cannot fail to be.

It is best for the assistant sister to spend all her time in the wards, the same as the staff nurses and probationers, except when absent for meals, or for her times off duty ; her daily " two hours off " should not be taken at the same time as the ward sister's, but at any other convenient part of the morning or afternoon.

Assistant sisters must be encouraged to specially interest themselves in the new probationers, and make it their business to impart to them without delay the rudiments of skilled nursing. For instance, between five and seven P.M. they should teach them how to make beds, by making the beds with them, and explaining the process as they do the work ; how to take temperatures ; how to read the measure glasses and many other details which need not be specified.

They should frequently impress upon beginners the importance of accuracy and thoroughness in performing every duty which falls to a nurse's share, and should never forget how much it lies in their power to give new-comers kindly encouragement, a true conception of the importance of strict obedience to rule, and a high standard of work from their first entrance into hospital life.

The dealings of assistant sisters with new probationers should not end there, but the ward sister should encourage them to compare notes with her as to their various characteristics, and so impress upon them, in every instance, the grave responsibility which devolves upon every experienced sister of forming a true estimate of the character and capabilities of each one sent to work under her.

Assistant sisters should perform any duty allotted to them, whether incidentally or regularly, by the sister under whom they are serving, and, when not otherwise engaged, they should help the staff nurses and probationers in the discharge of their ordinary duties, and gather up all the knowledge they can from the many sources open to them.

If assistant sisters reflect on their position and

prospects, they can scarcely fail to make the most of their invaluable opportunities for acquiring a thorough knowledge of the principles of practical supervision and ward management. They should cultivate a habit of careful observation, paying special attention to such points as are considered mere drudgery by unconscientious workers, and should never forget that the knowledge and experience they are making their own will result in increased capacity for taking a fuller measure of responsibility in due course.

A nurse who is promoted to be an assistant sister should keep three objects steadily before her in her daily work, and the sister under whom she is studying should never allow her to lose sight of them.

1st. It is her chief business to acquire a thorough knowledge of what is expected from those filling responsible posts.

2nd. To teach others what she has already been taught herself.

3rd. To make her "assistance" of such a quality that it cannot fail to be of present value to all with whom she is brought in contact, as well as a true and faithful preparation for future responsibilities.

Ward sisters and night sisters—for assistant sisters should, when possible, learn the respective duties by serving under both—may sometimes forget the importance of their influence over their subordinates, but they can scarcely fail to perceive their grave responsibility when they are directly preparing others to fill positions similar to their own. Those who have true enthusiasm for their work will inspire every pupil with some degree of the same, and rejoice to find that their experience has borne some fruit which they can gather for the benefit of others.

It is of immense value to those who have to teach to have the *possibilities* of their work clearly placed before them, and it is not fair either to the work, or to the individual, to leave each new-comer to discover these entirely for themselves.

Each one will have to learn by her own experience in many respects, however ready others may be to help her, but this fact should not deter those, who have gone through the same ordeal, from rendering all the generous aid to beginners which may be in their power.

No high-minded worker would wish to see her own errors repeated, especially if she realises that it rests with her in some measure to prevent this.

Those sisters who have made the best use of their own opportunities, will have learnt to estimate to some extent the value of example ; and the knowledge that the next generation of workers is prepared to accept their standard as its own, cannot fail to inspire the noblest natures with the desire to correct their own shortcomings, and to endeavour with renewed zeal to develop into that type of sister which they would desire to see those become, who are destined to follow in their steps.

CHAPTER VI.

OUR next consideration, and the most important to which we have yet turned our attention, is the relationship of the sister to her patients, and happily this is the chief attraction of her work.

But for the patients, no hospital sisters would need to exist, and with many the desire to nurse the sick and injured has probably been the principal motive in seeking this position.

The patients are interesting to a sister from two or three points of view. There is the broad human interest of their individual lives, various as they are in external circumstances and personal character. There is the unrivalled opportunity of learning what life means in many different aspects outside the walls of a hospital, to that class from which the majority of the patients come. The most indefatigable district visitor will but rarely have a glimpse of the inner life of those she calls upon, in the same way that it constantly reveals itself in the wards. To begin with, the patients are at home with each other in a sense in which they can but seldom feel equally at their ease with even a kindly outsider of another social rank. They may speak of themselves and of

(144)

their troubles with every appearance of candour and every desire to be candid, when questioned by a skilful and sympathetic visitor, and occasionally with a clear result. But the picture of their daily lives presented by their friendly talks with their social equals, as to their weekly wages and manner of spending them, what constitutes pleasure to them, and what their disappointments consist of, these—and a hundred details of similar nature—are infinitely more graphic than any impression that can be gained under ordinary circumstances. The experience which a sister acquires in this manner is valuable in many ways. Her sympathies can scarcely fail to be much enlarged by what she hears and sees, and the insight into the wants and wishes and troubles of her patients, which she will gradually possess from association with them, will immensely increase her power of helping them.

It is difficult to serve people effectually when we are very much in the dark as to their real needs, and it is a distinct aid towards understanding individuals, if we have obtained a thorough insight into the views and habits of the class to which they belong. As an illustration of this, we may take the first impression that any sympathetic visitor to a hospital will almost invariably receive, and which finds expression in some such exclamation as : " How dreadful it must be to be amongst so many people when one is ill ! *I* should long to be alone ! " Sister generally smiles when she hears this remark, knowing well that her patients almost invariably prefer being with others,

and that if the nature of their illness necessitates
that they should be placed in a separate room for a
time, they are nearly always anxious to get back to
the ward again, complaining that they "feel lonely"
and "want more company". Of course there are
exceptions to this, but the preference for being
together is distinctly the general rule.

It is obvious that we must understand their likes
and dislikes before we can make such arrangements
as are likely to contribute to their comfort socially,
and most of us will have discovered during our
training, that many of our preconceived notions as
to the patients, and their probable wants, were far
removed from the reality. One of the many advantages incidental to hospital work is, that it helps us
to get rid of inaccurate ideas upon many subjects,
and brings us face to face with facts as they are, and
not as we imagine them to be.

One of the most satisfactory conclusions that long
experience of all sorts of patients brings to the
majority of sisters is that human nature is worthy
of greater respect and admiration than they had
previously believed. They have experienced a genuine
surprise again and again, during their nursing career,
at the heroic endurance, and brave self-restraint and
self-denial in acute suffering, which they have
occasionally witnessed in men, women, and children;
and in this way many sisters will have been impressed anew with the truly grand capabilities of
that human nature which they share. It is much to
be able to say this amidst abundant evidence, on the

other hand, of all that is low, degrading, and repulsive; and perhaps a cursory observer might only be aware of the equally true and most deplorable side of life, which is but too sadly represented in the wards of a hospital. Nevertheless, even those who are not much given to see below the surface of what takes place before them, will often involuntarily bear testimony to their deepening appreciation of the noble qualities that manifest themselves in directions where one might least expect to find them.

It is a great encouragement to know that those who have worked the longest, and seen the most, are the most cognisant of the ennobling influence which their work has a tendency to produce upon their sympathies and general views of life.

If the tendency of hospital work were to make earnest workers less hopeful, it would be a very discouraging element to take into consideration in resolving to devote oneself to it. But we are enabled to persevere with renewed confidence, if those who are best qualified to speak, are able to tell us, from their own practical experience, that the reverse of this is the case.

I have referred to this because we are sometimes slow to perceive that we are gaining any personal advantage from our dealings with the patients, but now we have chiefly to consider what the sister can do for them.

To begin with, what kind of a welcome awaits them when they are first brought to the ward? I fear that comparatively few sisters attach sufficient importance to this detail.

To them the arrival of a new patient is a very ordinary occurrence, and they fail to remember that it is probably a unique experience to each individual patient. They smile good-naturedly when the patient has become happy and contented in his new surroundings, and has confided to them the relief he or she feels in finding the hospital " so comfortable," and everybody " so kind," when they " couldn't bear the thought of coming in to begin with," and feared the hospital would prove a " dreadful place ". This oft-repeated tale might surely teach those who are familiar with it, what need there is for a friendly reception, when the reluctant patient is brought to their ward. It must be remembered that they are not only strange, but ill, and very often in actual pain, so that they are not in a normal condition for going through the ordeal of being consigned into strange hands, and, unless they are too ill to take any notice, which, of course, frequently happens, the way they are spoken to, on their first arrival, will make a wonderful difference to them. In the worst cases, when the patient is apparently beyond the influence of kindly words, the anxious friends who have brought him will be eager and grateful for them. They will leave the patient with the burden of their great anxiety lightened or increased, very much in accordance with what has been said or left unsaid, apart from what may actually have been done for him. It is true that the feeling of strangeness soon passes away, but, as it is painful while it lasts, it is well worth while to shorten it as much as possible. The patient has been sent to the ward, which implies that he is in need of help, and that the doctor intends to see what can be done for him. The hospital has provided every means possible for relieving his distress and adding to his comfort, and surely it rests with the sister to dispeuse the hospitality which is placed, as it were, at her disposal, in a manner which shall make it most acceptable to the recipient. That many sisters possess the kindly feeling which would dispose them to do this, no one who knows them could question for a moment, and the lamentable failure to give any evidence of it, which exists in so many cases, may probably be attributed to a want of perception that the need is very great in the first instance, and that it rests with them to supply it in the second. Of course a busy sister cannot always be free to say to every new patient the few kindly words that constitute an important part of the welcome given, but this is another point which she must impress upon her nurses by constant precept and unwearied example, whenever it happens that she is free to attend personally to this duty.

The test of a sister's management is not so much whether everything is as it should be in her wards, when she is present to secure it, but whether the same can be said when she is not there, or, in other words, whether she can ensure that her wishes are carried out habitually in such details as are of neces-

sity executed by other hands. What a sister can
actually *do* in this and other matters is, or should be,
comparatively little to what she can *get done* by
exerting her legitimate influence in the various
directions where its effect could be traced with
advantage. No one familiar with the actual work
that is always going on in a large ward could wonder
that the welcome to each patient, which to an outsider seems a matter of course, should constantly be
omitted as a matter of fact, by those to whom the
arrival of a new patient, or, it may be of many new
patients at the same time, forms a mere incident in
the day's routine. It would be utterly unreasonable
to say that there is no excuse for a sister, whose
mind is occupied with a dozen important items at
the same time, if she ignores the existence of a new
patient until there is something actually to be done
for him, but if her sympathy is sufficiently active to
realise what the process of arriving means to a large
proportion of new patients, she will take care that
those whose business it is to put them to bed, and
attend to their immediate wants, shall have some
conception of the trial that it probably is to them, and
some knowledge of the best means to soften it, by
kindly words and manner in the midst of the work.
We know that the patient will shortly be much
more comfortable, but this is a fact which *he* has
yet to realise, and that makes a considerable difference for the time. The most trivial expressions
to the effect that he will shortly feel more at home,
gentle inquiries as to the nature or length of the

illness, if the patient appears in a condition to like answering the questions, and does not seem to find it an effort to do so ; indeed, any manifestation of individual interest which may suggest itself at the moment, will meet with a quick response.

Nothing but a *habit* of showing this helpful interest will ensure some evidence of it on all occasions, and I am confident that many nurses would be at the pains of cultivating it, if they once realised what it means to the patient. I would not be misunderstood to suggest a noisy, chattering welcome from nurses to patients. Even silence would often be less worrying than anything so supremely undesirable and un-nurse-like as that. Half-a-dozen words conveying the right meaning would often be all that is needed, but let us remember that these *are* needed. If the nurse has in her mind the idea of showing hospitality, that is the chief point. Her own tact and ever-increasing experience will teach her what is the most fitting manifestation of it in each instance.

A sister who sees one patient after another arriving, when her wards are already filled with extra beds, may well be forgiven for feeling too worried in arranging what to do with the fresh arrivals, to have any kind words to spare for them ; indeed, she exhibits an amount of self-control which may well command our admiration, if she refrains from impatient exclamations at their appearance, and from giving short answers to the nurses who besiege her in all directions to know what is to be done, when she feels that *that* is about the last thing she is able to tell them ! The difficulties are often so numerous and perplexing that we cannot feel disposed to blame a sister, who is honestly doing her best for all concerned, if she has become oblivious of the feelings of those who are dependent upon her. It would be well if she could remember amidst the temporary confusion—or the nearest approach to that state which it is possible for a pressure of work to create in a well-organised ward—that the mere fact of additional patients being sent up, when the beds are already full, indicates that the cases are probably in greater need of help than usual; that they are not clay figures, but human beings, keenly alive to all that is taking place, especially to the fact that they are not wanted, as that is what affects them personally more than anything else. If it were possible for the sister to retain a consciousness of all this, amidst the other practical considerations that are pressing upon her for the moment, she would gain a still higher step in that calmness of demeanour, and that unruffled self-control, which some sisters already possess in an admirable degree. There is much excuse for her if she cannot attain to this; but, if she recognises that the omission needs an excuse, a distinct advance will have been made towards the perfection which is here indicated, as a very difficult, but not impossible standard.

The patients' friends are generally less attractive than the patients themselves, as the latter call out our sympathies by claiming our help, whereas the former sometimes contrive to make themselves very troublesome indeed. Nothing but tact, and the know-

ledge of how best to deal with them which comes by
experience, can teach the sister the wisest and kindest
manner of replying to their anxious and innumerable
questions. She should make a point of seeing as
much as she can of the patients' friends on visiting
days, giving them all, as far as possible, a chance of
speaking to her if they wish it. If they have any
grievance, real or imaginary, they are much more
likely to complain, and so make a remedy or explanation possible, than if they feel there is no connection
between them and the sister, as they naturally will do,
if she fails to display any interest in them. Some
sisters, because they are conscious of feeling a kindly
regard for the patients and their affairs, expect them
and their friends to realise this without any sort of
indication or expression of it, but this is scarcely
reasonable.

Confidence on the part of the patients and their
friends in the sister's kindness and judgment is of
the greatest service in dealing with them. They
will probably be more straightforward, in many
instances, about that difficult matter for supervision
every visiting day, the bringing in of all sorts of
unwholesome provisions to patients whose condition
sometimes makes the viands a source of positive
danger. Tact and discrimination will go a long
way towards keeping the peace, and soothing the
injured feelings that the well-advised prohibition is
apt to create. Great firmness is essential. Only
those experienced in such matters can form any
conception of the amount and variety of the food

brought in for the patients of all ages by their well-meaning, but ignorant friends.   A collection of what has to be confiscated in a single set of wards on one visiting day is sometimes a curious sight.   Lockers, and occasionally beds, have to be searched to prevent the patients swallowing what would do them harm in proportion to the pernicious character of the food, and their unfavourable condition for receiving it. Nevertheless, it is for the sister to exercise common-sense in the application of the rule which forbids provisions to be brought in to patients.   If harmless extras are brought by the friends, it is much better for the sister to allow them to be kept, pending the doctor's decision as to whether the patient may safely indulge in them or not, than to insist upon their removal as a matter of routine, regardless of the comfort and satisfaction of the individual case. Stimulants of all kinds are, of course, strictly for-bidden.   In some cases every description of solid food would he harmful, but there are many others when wholesome food might safely be permitted, if the doubtful articles were brought openly to the sister, for her to ascertain from the doctor, when next he visits the ward, if he will allow the patient to partake of them.

This is not a matter to leave to the staff nurse. She has no authority to sanction any infringement of a rule made for the general good, however desirable it may appear to be, but she can always fall back upon the fact that sister may be asked about it, if the friends are inclined to resent what they may probably deem too rigid an enforcement of the regulation. They are all inclined to regard their own case as an exception, but a sister will best judge when such an exception may be judiciously asked for, and will endeavour that a wise application of the rule shall supersede its indiscriminate enforcement. The regulation is manifestly made for the patient's own good, and it is one that is best fulfilled to the spirit rather than to the letter. If any practical difficulty arises, there is the rule, known to all, to which the sister can appeal, but my experience is that she will have less trouble in making her authority felt, in cases where it becomes necessary to speak and act firmly, if she places an intelligent interpretation on the standing order, and thus complies with the real wishes of the authorities in this matter. A rule intended to exclude stimulants, marvellous compounds *called* cakes, puddings, and pies, etc. (though showing no other resemblance to the articles we usually associate with these names!), need not in some cases necessarily exclude wholesome biscuits, the few little acid drops that some patients treasure up carefully to take after their medicine, or perhaps fresh country eggs. If the general feeling is that sister would like the patients to have anything that is good for them, they will, on the whole, be more straightforward, and accept her decision in these matters with less reluctance.

It is very important occasionally that the sister should know how to extract from the patient's friends such information as the doctors may wish to possess, and which it is often impossible to obtain from the

patient himself. Doctors and sisters know what a
tax upon time and patience has frequently to be paid
before the desired *facts* can be elicited, and sometimes
considerable skill is required to eliminate these from
the voluminous and unimportant statements with
which they are mixed up. An intelligent sister can
prove very useful in this direction, both in conversa-
tions with the patients, and with their friends on
visiting days. It is curious to notice how readily a
patient will confide troubles and interests of all sorts
to a sister who has once won his confidence, and the
sister who hears the most is generally one whose interest in her patients places more means at her disposal
for helping them in various ways.

This power of sympathising with many opposite
temperaments under many varied circumstances is a
gift which we possess in very different degrees, and
some really kind-hearted people appear to have a very
small share of it. It must be conceded that great
efforts in this direction will sometimes produce only
limited results. Yet, the fact remains, that it is
important that the exceptional openings afforded by
hospital work for the cultivation and exercise of this
helpful gift should be recognised, so that those who
have only one talent may do their utmost with it, and
that those who are more favoured may exert themselves to the full extent of their power and opportunity.

It is difficult enough for a sister to find or make
time for much conversation with her patients beyond
that which is confined to their immediate needs.

That an immense field for useful influence lies in this direction is sufficiently obvious, but it must be left for each individual sister to cultivate it as seems to her best. If she feels that nurses have some work to do in this way for their patients, and that their physical necessities cannot be altogether separated from their other not less real, if less tangible, requirements, she will do what she can to meet *all* their needs, even more by making others see and help them, than she can possibly do herself in the midst of her multifarious duties. "If thou draw out thy *soul* to the hungry and satisfy the afflicted soul, then shall thy light rise in obscurity and thy darkness be as the noonday." The amount that some sisters accomplish in this way, in addition to all their other work, sometimes appears marvellous, and is noteworthy as an encouraging example for others. In many ways it must bring them a great reward, and it cannot but call forth our cordial admiration.

The responsibility of deciding whether the condition of the patient renders it desirable for his name to be added to the "dangerous list" does not finally rest with the sister, but this is, nevertheless, a matter in which her suggestions have considerable influence, and upon which she has frequently to bestow a great deal of anxious thought. There are often many conflicting interests to be taken into consideration— the welfare of the patient, his wishes and the anxiety of the friends—who, in many of these cases, will soon be left to mourn their loss. It is not always easy to know how to get this matter arranged for the

best, even with the kindest intentions to all concerned. The sister, or the nurse has the first opportunity of noting any sudden change that has occurred;
therefore it rests with her to ascertain the doctor's
views on this question directly it appears to be
necessary, unless he places the matter beyond doubt
by saying at once what he wishes to be done about
it. Often the only "friends" in existence, or available, are the kind of people that appear sadly out of
place near a sick or dying person. On the other
hand, we must remember that the companionship of
the least satisfactory of old friends, or even a mere
acquaintance who is associated with the former life
of a patient, may be more acceptable to him than
the utmost kindness from those in the hospital, if he
has only come there "at the last" and they are
strangers to him. We must not forget that the
desirability of the friends' presence depends much
more upon the patient's feelings with regard to them,
than upon the impression they make upon us. The
familiar sight of what appears to us a very unattractive, not to say repulsive figure, the harsh sound of
a very gruff voice uttering words, that to our ears
are not very tender, or even kindly, the heavy footfall
of most ungainly boots, may be eagerly listened for
and welcomed by the patient, and may do more to
diminish the terrible sense of loneliness that is creep-
ing over him, than our gentlest and most sweetly
expressed sympathy could do. We do well to be
aware of this fact, not with the thought of making
our attentions less effective, but so that we may know

the relative importance to the patient of what can be done to soothe the entrance into the dark valley, apart from the actual ministrations to his physical need that it rests with us to render.

The points which must influence a sister, as far as the dangerous list question rests with her, are, " Will it be any comfort or satisfaction to the patient to feel that the ' friends ' are near him ? and will it be some consolation to the friends, when all is over, to have had every opportunity of what they graphically term ' seeing the last of him ' ? " Of course, I do not mean that these reflections have anything to do with obeying the standing orders of the institution on the subject, but it is obviously desirable that the sister should not lose sight of these considerations in connection with the carrying out of the regulations. If a patient dies without being " on the dangerous list," as we know must sometimes be the case in spite of every precaution that could possibly have been taken to prevent it, one cannot but feel that, while it is an incident that creates a natural regret at the time, the recollection of it, provided no one is to blame for the omission, soon passes away, but, to the relatives of the deceased, it *may* be an addition to their sorrow that will add to the weight of it all the rest of their lives. I know that often this might not be the case, but then the mere possibility of it is very serious.

Neglect in this respect goes far to create a prejudice against hospitals, which is unfair to them on the one hand, and not kind to the class of people for whom they exist on the other, as they can but leave their sick in these institutions when they have not adequate means to provide for them at home. It is superfluous that this terrible dread of any difficulty about visiting at critical seasons, should add to the anxiety of those who have brought the patient to the hospital, or should, perhaps, even altogether deter a sick person from entering an institution to seek the aid that might in some cases save life, and in others, at least, alleviate suffering. I do not say that this result inevitably follows, but those who have observed the power of prejudice, and the difficulty of over- coming it, will be aware that the risk of these ignorant prejudices being increased by facts of this kind is not exaggerated.

There is a sense of utter desolation connected with the idea of dying alone in the wards of a hospital—that is to say, separated from all who have a personal interest in the sufferer, notwith- standing that kind hands may be doing all that strangers can to soften the final trial, and when friends exist, it is worth a great deal of trouble on the part of the sister and others to enable them to be present. The sorrow is inevitable, but the one consolation the bereaved friends can have, at the time, lies in the fact, so often expressed amidst tears to the sister or nurse, "Everything has been done for him ; you have all been so good and so kind; I *know* nothing else could have been done!" Let us give the mourners this comfort at any rate. The knowledge that they are *able* to do so is one of the sweetest compensations sisters and nurses meet with in their work.

One of the hardest things that a sister has to do is to break the news of an unexpected death to sorrowing relatives, especially if they are totally unprepared for the shock awaiting them. It is a great temptation to leave this painful task to any one else who can be found to fulfil it, but the knowledge that the very sympathy which makes her dread to undertake it will, probably, enable her to do it more kindly than one who felt less reluctance to go through the distressing scene, will nerve an earnest sister to carry out this duty. In the presence of great sorrow nothing that can be said or done will seem to alleviate it at first, but it will help more than it appears to do even at the time, and everything that sister can tell them about the end of their beloved relative will be treasured up and thought of afterwards. All that could possibly give any comfort should be detailed at length, and all questions patiently answered, while the relation of such incidents as could but be painful in remembrance may well be spared the mourners, or passed over as lightly as circumstances permit. "We want people to feel with us more than to act for us," as George Eliot says, and this is a fact that we should keep before us, especially at a time when nothing we can *do* is likely to be of any avail, and what our sympathy may prompt us to *say* may prove a real source of consolation.

It is hardly possible to judge of the extent of the grief felt, by the outward expression of it. Some take the sad news quietly because they are heart-

11

broken; some are stupefied, as it were, at the terrible
intelligence, and too overwhelmed to collect their
thoughts, or to know what to do or say next; and
others, of whom we meet too many in a hospital,
are simply indifferent. Some, again, are extremely
demonstrative, and give way to every external
symptom of grief that occurs to them, which, I
think, does not indicate that they are suffering
either more or less than those who bear their sorrow
in comparative silence, but merely that it is the
manner of expression natural to them in a condition
of great trouble and excitement. There is no form
of comfort that can be recommended for universal
application, but a kind sister, knowing that very
little *can* be done, will do that little as unselfishly
as she can. Fortunately, this sad side of her work
is by no means that which claims the largest share
of her time and attention, but only one of the calls
for self-sacrifice which she must be prepared to meet
bravely when they occur.

I have not spoken of the special nursing duties
connected with the patients, for that, being the
primary object of a sister's attention, is not likely
to be lost sight of, and is a portion of hospital work
too wide and complete in itself to be entered upon
here. The interest of the " case " is far less likely
to be overlooked than the interest in the " patient,"
and an intelligent sister will seldom ignore the
opportunities of increasing the knowledge of her
profession which her position affords. As she is
a teacher of others, she must lose no opportunity of

learning herself. The variety of cases and new modes of treatment, that are always to be found in the wards of a busy hospital, are full of instruction for those who are able and desirous of profiting by them. Probationers will not notice symptoms, or have any idea of their relative importance with a view to reporting them to the doctor at once, or of waiting for his regular visit, until the sister has pointed them out; and before she can do this she will necessarily be obliged to observe them herself, or, at any rate, to know something about them. In teaching others a sister will find how much and how little she knows—two points that she can but ascertain with advantage. Probationers will ask many questions of a sister, who has the patience of a good teacher, that she may not know how to answer. It is best to say at once that she is not able to explain, but, if it is a sensible question, a clever sister will not fail to seize the very first opportunity of improving her own and the probationer's mind on that subject. A sister may rightly object to being asked questions at inconvenient times and places; but if she has occasion to reprove a nurse or probationer for so doing, she should make it very clear that it is not the fact of being asked questions that she complains of, but the inopportune moment that has been chosen for the purpose. The asking of intelligent questions is a habit to be distinctly encouraged on all matters connected with the study of nursing.

It is a duty that a sister owes to her patients to keep herself well up in all knowledge that can by any possibility be of practical use to them in her work. She has so many opportunities of adding to the nursing knowledge that it was essential for her to acquire as a qualification for her post, that there is little excuse for the indifference to progress, which alone could explain her making no further advancement.

Besides, a sister should not forget that she has to make herself in every way competent to be an efficient help to the doctors in carrying out the treatment they prescribe. I am assuming that every sister has been sufficiently well grounded in the rudiments of her work for it to be unnecessary for me to remind her that *obedience to orders* is one of her fundamental claims to being considered a " trained nurse ".

But no good sister will feel that her training is ever finished, more particularly as it applies to her powers of observation, and of reporting to the doctor. Her value to him, and therefore to the patients, will be immensely enhanced by her skill in these respects; and she should continue to cultivate this industriously. *How* to observe as well as what to observe, and how to convey the result of her observations to the doctor in concise language, and in a manner calculated to give him a clear and full statement of the facts he is seeking to ascertain, is a matter worthy of much painstaking on the part of the sister. To help the doctor, not to add to his difficulties, is the object a hospital sister has to keep in view. A greater knowledge of the patient's wishes, circumstances, and other personal matters, as well as of the facts connected with his illness, would often be of service to the doctor, and it is disappointing if his inquiries fail to elicit the information he desires. Some sisters take sufficient interest to *know* all these things, but take no pains to acquire a business-like manner of conveying the information to the doctor. The patients can but suffer from this awkward reticence, and every sister should make an effort to report, and to answer questions, accurately and intelligently.

One of the difficulties awaiting every sister is having to deal with the complaints of patients against nurses, and of nurses against patients, which are certain to arise from time to time. A great deal of tact is frequently required to settle these little grievances. One point the sister must insist upon, *i.e.*, that she will not permit any quarrelling between nurses and patients. Whatever the complaint is, it must be brought to her to settle, for she is in a better position to judge of the merits of the case than those whose feelings are disturbed by the incident under discussion. The patient will often listen to the sister, if she knows how to speak firmly to him, when he would only become more and more offensive to the nurse, if the difference between them is allowed to develop into a dispute. There are patients who behave intolerably in spite of every consideration and kindness, but extreme insubordination would ensure the discharge of such. Many nurses are exceedingly forbearing with the most irritating and ungrateful of patients, but some, on the other hand, find it hard to make sufficient allowance for the rudeness with which they are occasionally greeted, when they are striving to do their duty.

The sister must encourage her nurses to be very gentle and patient, very charitable in the excuses that can be made by their kindness for conduct that, in itself, appears inexcusable. Whilst doing this on the one hand, she must speak very decidedly to the patients on the other, and clearly give them to understand that they are not expected to take advantage of nurse's kindness. They will listen to sister when they would have quarrelled with nurse many a time. If the sister insists upon having the beginning of the misunderstanding reported to her, she will often be able to prevent little scenes, the memory of which would interfere with the patient's comfort during the rest of his stay in the hospital, or, perhaps, predispose him to leave it earlier than is desirable. As a rule, nurses are wonderfully patient and forbearing, but there are occasions when they are more to blame than the ignorant, suffering patients, who are behaving badly. At the same time there is much to try a nurse's powers of endurance beyond ordinary limits, and a little opportune sympathy from sister will help her to go on cheerfully.

When a patient complains of some neglect, such as the failure to give a medicine that is rightly due, or inattention to his real wants, the sister must have no hesitation in speaking to the nurse on the subject. It need scarcely be said that no one would find fault

with a person in the presence of others without some
necessity for so doing, but while some sisters, with
uncontrolled tempers, fail to remember this, others
have a sort of idea that no nurse must be blamed in
the presence of a patient; and that is simply absurd.
If a nurse has put on a fomentation in such a way as
to make the patient's bed thoroughly wet and uncomfortable, if, in short, anything has been done for him
in an unskilled manner, or if some treatment that he
should have received has been overlooked, the sister
should call the nurse's attention to the matter *in
the presence of the patient,* and see that the cause of
complaint is remedied. I do not mean that she need
scold the nurse, but that she should speak of the
deficiency at once, and let the patient have the
satisfaction of feeling that he is sure of attention
and justice while under sister's care. I have known
nurses entertain the most ridiculous ideas on this point,
and take refuge in a fit of sulkiness, retire in tears,
or answer the sister rudely, because they "cannot be
spoken to before the patient". It never seems to
occur to them that while it is for the sister to support
them when they are right, it is certainly not for her
to uphold them when they are wrong!

A sister need not blame her nurses before the
patients for defects of which the latter are not conscious, and she must be careful to ascertain that the
complaint is just, reproving the patient if it is not.
But the sooner she clears up her nurses' minds on
the point of her right to speak to them whenever she
sees the necessity, the better it will be. It requires

more moral courage on the part of the sister than the nurses have any idea of sometimes, but the sister must inspire nurses and patients with confidence in her justice, and she will fail to do this if she apparently ignores what she perceives to be a reasonable ground for complaint.　There are many exceptions ; but a sister will find in the long run that patients are slow to complain, unless when roused by an irritating manner, or if they chance to have a passionate temper. As a rule, they are more likely to refrain from speaking when they have cause, than to speak without, alleging if inquiries are made that they " do not like to get nurse into trouble ".　It is for the sister to try to be perfectly fair to both, and to make both aware that this is her desire.

Another matter which the sister should make a point of keeping in her own hands is the decision whether patients shall be allowed to get up for an hour or two in the morning to help with the early morning work.　Nurses will be scrupulously careful in keeping patients in bed when they are not allowed to get up at all ; but many of them appear to think that directly a patient is " ordered up " for an hour or two in the evening, they may be expected to help in the same way as patients who are up for half the day, and who are quite strong enough for the exertion. I do not wish to imply that nurses are actually un-kind enough to insist upon patients doing what they have not sufficient strength for, but hospital sisters are aware that many nurses are apt to be thoughtless in this respect.　They will either ask a patient to get up, or yield to his not infrequent desire to do more than is good for him in the way of helping, as soon as the doctor's sanction to his beginning to "get about again" has once been obtained. In some cases there is no possible objection to this; but to ensure a careful judgment in the matter, the sister should insist that the nurse refers to her in each instance, before a patient is allowed to get up and help with the morning work.

The recreation for the patients, of a kind adapted to their individual tastes and condition, is another detail that claims the sister's attention, and one in which she should encourage her nurses to interest themselves. Many of them will like reading, but they will probably wait for it to be suggested to them before they ask for a book. It is worth a little trouble to see that a patient who is able to amuse himself in this way has the kind of book likely to suit him. Some of them enjoy games of draughts, dominoes, or other amusements of this kind. Women are usually glad to occupy themselves with a little needlework, if the nature of their illness permits them to pass the time in this way, but they will probably need some one to produce it, with a question as to their feeling inclined to do it. Much depends upon making the long hours pass as cheerfully as possible, and this cannot be done without constant trouble. The days are very monotonous to those who can only hope to get well slowly, and who can count the length of their sojourn in the hospital by many weeks.

The right kind of visitor from outside will receive

an eager welcome ; her presence has the brightening effect of a breath of fresh air upon those who have become weary in the hospital atmosphere. It is of great value to those who are well enough for it, to see any one who has time and patience to *listen* to them, and who can give them something new to think about. Sisters should realise the importance of variety and change in the mental surroundings of their patients, and procure it for them as much as they can.

Nevertheless, ward visitors, who are not of the right sort, often tax a sister's patience very severely, and contrive to add to her anxieties by their want of tact. The sister must ensure that every kind of visitor receives courtesy in her wards, and remember that giving outsiders a pleasant impression, and an insight into the varied needs of her patients, is one of the duties of her position that she is not free to ignore.

Much of the success of the ward visitor will depend upon the sister, although there are some well-meaning persons so devoid of tact, and so unsuited for the task they have undertaken, that nothing can make their visits otherwise than unsatisfactory.

An experienced sister soon perceives whether her visitor is really desirous of doing her chosen work in a pleasant, business-like way, or whether visits to the hospital have been taken up temporarily for the mere charm of novelty. All fresh visitors should, at any rate, have the benefit of the doubt, and not be discouraged from what is to many of them quite a formidable undertaking in the first instance, by the reception they meet with from the sister and her nurses.

It is best for the sister to frankly explàin to a new-comer under what conditions her visits will be cor-dially welcome. If a visitor understood from the first that, if doctors enter the ward, hospital etiquette demands that she should immediately leave it while they are in possession, the chances are that the visitor will not need to have her attention called to this a second time. The sister should point out also where the visitor can take refuge during this temporary in-terruption, for if the visits take place on days selected for the purpose, the stay of the doctors would not in all probability be of long duration, as they would not then be making their regular round of the wards. A hint pleasantly given that ward visitors have been known to read or talk in a very loud tone of voice, when physicians or surgeons are busy in the adjoining ward, and that this cannot be permitted, may prevent a repetition of this offence, and the consequent ne-cessity of requiring the fresh visitor to desist.

Then again, some indirect guidance upon the point of how much or how little the visitor is expected to see of the sister, would be acceptable to those who sincerely wish to do the right thing, and who yet are naturally puzzled, in conditions entirely new to them, to know what the right thing is. I feel great sym-pathy with a sister who, in the midst of many anxieties, is afflicted with a fussy visitor all the after-noon, but I have also had reason to deplore the want of that sympathetic perception which should enable

her to put herself, as it were, in the stranger's place,
and not expect *all* the consideration to come from
one unfamiliar with life inside a hospital, and, therefore, ignorant, rather than unmindful, of a sister's
special trials and difficulties!

" I should like Miss —— so much if she would only
visit my patients instead of devoting all her time to
me!" said a cheerful, busy sister the other day and
I have no doubt that this sentiment would have been
echoed all round, if it had been uttered in the presence
of many sisters.

If the sister happens to be disengaged when the
visitor arrives, let her welcome her cordially, and tell
her anything of special interest concerning any patient
whom she may know, or be going to see, but having
done that, and seen her visitor fairly started with the
patients, the sister has done all that can reasonably
be expected of her. If the sister is engaged when the
visitor arrives, let the nurse in the ward be ready to
receive the visitor pleasantly, and let the sister see
her for a minute or two when she is free to do so.
But, if it sometimes happens, as it well may do in our
busy wards, that the sister is fully engaged the whole
afternoon, the visitor need not feel herself slighted,
nor the sister feel that she has neglected a duty, if the
tone of the wards is such as to ensure order and
courtesy throughout. On the next occasion the sister
would doubtless endeavour to see a little more of her
visitor, but she should not hesitate to say if necessary,
that she is more busy than she appears to be, if she
has duties to perform from which she has been un-

duly hindered. The main point is to establish an easy relationship between the head of a ward and any regular visitor. The latter should be made to feel that she can mention any little difficulty she has met with, or any trifling complaint that has been poured into her ears, without fear of giving offence, or stirring up strife. In most cases a word of explanation will suffice to clear away any misrepresentation. It is much better that this should be said to the sister herself, than that a wrong impression should be spread outside the hospital, and this would not infrequently happen if the sister is unapproachable. On the other hand, most sisters know the comfort of having a kind friend for their patients, who is often able, as well as ready and willing, to help them in a variety of ways impossible to the sister herself. Many a case of heart-rending distress receives the form of relief best adapted to its need through the lady visitor, many a weary hour is brightened by the fresh interests she brings into sad lives, that are never so conscious of their own dreariness as when lying through long days or weeks with nothing to lift them out of themselves, or to help them to escape from the memory of their personal worries and troubles. A sister, with a motherly love for her patients in her heart, will note, with approval, faces light up in welcome greeting of the popular and expected ward visitor, and she would do her best to secure this relief and pleasure for them, even if it involved greater personal trouble to herself than, strictly speaking, need be the case. The circumstances which demand that the sister's time and attention should be devoted to a ward visitor for any considerable part of an afternoon must be very exceptional, and both sister and visitor should learn to recognise this. Most visitors would resent the notion, if it once occurred to them, that they visited a ward to be " entertained " by a busy sister, who, being " on duty," has a dozen legitimate claims upon her time and attention. Without ignoring the courtesy due on either side, a true view of the mutual relations of a sister and her ward visitor would tend to simplify matters very much.

As I have previously said, there is scarcely any limit to the demands that the patients make upon a good sister. They need, and for the most part will gratefully accept, every sort of help that she can give or procure them. Hospital sisters can fully realise the truth of Miss Proctor's words :—

> " And as material life is planned
> That even the loneliest one must stand
> Dependent on his brother's hand ;
> So links more subtle and more fine
> Bind every other soul to thine
> In one great brotherhood Divine ".

CHAPTER VII.

NIGHT SISTERS.—FINAL DETAILS.

As yet I have said nothing about the work of night sisters, or of the relationship which they and ward sisters bear to each other.

There is much need to understand the points of resemblance and the points of difference in the work allotted to each, as there is room for mutual helpfulness, and indeed a constant necessity for it. There is nothing in the nature of their respective duties to engender rivalry; and misunderstandings, which may arise without care, should be studiously avoided for the sake of the common work, which cannot but suffer if they occur.

The night sister's object is to help the day sister by giving the supervision to her patients and nurses, which the latter cannot exercise both night and day. Fortunately, much less attention is required in each set of wards at night than is essential for efficient management during the day, but this fact in itself may prove a source of difficulty, if the night sister has any tendency to be officious. On the other hand, very serious responsibility rests with the night sister, and she must have no hesitation in exercising her authority from fear of giving offence, if the exigencies of the work appear to demand it.

At one time any trustworthy person was considered competent to walk through a hospital as night superintendent, the chief duty attached to her appointment being to see that the nurses were awake, and apparently attending to their duties in their own wards, instead of wandering about the building, to the obvious neglect of their patients. Any knowledge of nursing, which could enable them to judge of the condition of the patients, or form any adequate idea as to the manner in which the various orders given for each case were being carried out by the nurses, was considered superfluous. Of late years this has entirely altered, and although the night sister is still responsible for the orderly conduct of nurses and wards during the night, this has become merely an incidental duty which she carries out as a matter of course, whilst discharging her duty towards the patients as far as circumstances will allow. The extent to which she is able to do this will depend considerably upon the clearness of the instructions and report left for her guidance by the day sister, as well as upon the capability of the night sister herself. The welfare of the patients for the time being must of necessity be much influenced by the degree of efficiency with which each sister enables the other to do her duty towards them.

The day sister should remember that she cannot easily estimate the anxiety of the night sister's position. She has to judge of the existing condition of the patient, with very little knowledge sometimes as to what may have taken place before. It is not enough to know that he is seriously ill, for that fact may be patent to the most casual observer; but the question is, " Is he worse than he has been during the day, or since the doctor last saw him?" If so, should the doctor be fetched to him, or what instructions have been left concerning the treatment, supposing a change for the worse to have been anticipated and to have taken place? The day sister will have had more opportunity of gathering the doctor's opinion, as well as of ascertaining his wishes, than the night sister *can* have, unless circumstances necessitate a special inquiry. This fact should convince the former of the desirability of giving as full information as possible concerning all that there is any probability of it being useful for the night sister to know.

Some sisters appear to think that as the night sister is responsible for many wards besides their own, it is not likely that she can bestow special attention upon any of their patients, and therefore they do not think it necessary to leave anything beyond the most meagre instructions for her. But this is not just towards patients or night sister. The greater the difficulties under which she is called upon to act, the more need for affording her all the help that can be given, and it is not fair to ignore the interest which a night sister may be expected to feel, because, it may be, she has not much chance of displaying it. The ward belongs, as it were, to the day sister, and though she is to some extent represented by the night sister for a few hours, the influence of her management is more or less supreme.

12

It may safely be predicted that the set of wards in which the night sister finds it easiest to do her duty, will be the one in which the good management reflects the most credit upon the day sister. It is both unkind and inefficient to create difficulties, or indeed not to take pains to remove them. Every good nurse is trained to make it easy for another to succeed her in charge of a patient, and to be able to give as full a report of the patient's symptoms and needs when occasion requires, as though no change of nurse had taken place. If this is incumbent upon those who are responsible for the nursing of an individual patient, the duty is not less on the part of those who have a large number of cases under their care. The sister's example in this respect will of course affect the conduct of her night nurses. She must make the orders concerning the patients, and any other instructions she may have to give, clear to the nurses. For any difficulty they may find in carrying out these orders, or for any additional instructions they may require, it is for them to apply to the night sister. It is their duty to report both to the night and to the day sister what may have taken place. If this is clearly understood and loyally enforced by each sister respectively, harmonious working will ensue throughout.

The night sister should be very slow to give any orders that would interfere with the directions of the day sister in reference to ward work, and should only do so when the immediate necessities of the patients appear to demand it. In case of this necessity it is well for the night sister to take an early opportunity of explaining what she has done, and why she thought it advisable, as it is over such incidents as these that matters are apt to get misrepresented, and a coldness springs up for which there is no real foundation. After all, a freedom from touchiness on both sides, and a prompt and straightforward explanation if such a course appear desirable to either, are the great points at which to aim, and it is only by conforming to the spirit thus indicated that a good practical result can be secured.

When I say that night sisters should not interfere with the day sister's wishes with regard to ward work, of course, I mean with individual arrangements, for both night and day sisters are equally bound to enforce the general regulations of the hospital to which they belong. For instance, night sisters must carefully insist that no ward breakfasts are served before 6 A.M., though they may be previously prepared and ready for distribution when the clock strikes. All general rules must be observed and enforced by the night as well as by the day sister. Indeed, anything short of this could not be considered conscientious service.

The warmth and ventilation of the wards should claim a due share of the night sister's attention; and as the airing of linen is carried out to a great extent on the lobbies between the wards at night, she should see that it is receiving proper care from the nurses, and that the guards have been left in place to prevent the possibility of accident.

A good night sister has it in her power to render useful help in all directions. She will endeavour to procure any instructions from the doctors, and ascertain their wishes in reference to any serious cases as far as possible before they retire for the night, so as to avoid calling them up unnecessarily. Of course, she will have no hesitation in disturbing them when the needs of the patients require it, for it would not be fair to them, neither could the doctors feel any confidence in a night sister, who did not appeal to them promptly when the necessity arose. There is all the difference between being called up in an emergency, and being roused up to answer a question that might easily have been asked before.

The question whether to call up a doctor or not is often one of great perplexity to a night sister. The wants of the patients must be placed first, and due attention to these should be combined with as much consideration as possible for every one else concerned.

One of the compensations for the perpetual anxieties of a night sister's post is the valuable experience in all kinds of cases, and the great variety of treatment and nursing with which her work renders her familiar. She cannot know as much of individual patients as their respective day sisters do; the number of the patients and the circumstances under which the night sister sees them preclude this possibility; but it is wonderful how much an intelligent night sister can learn about the cases, and the characters of the patients, if she is genuinely interested in them and her work, and knows how to elicit information from the nurses.

If the night sister recognises her place as a help to the day sister, whilst holding her own when occasion requires it, the report of how any special case may have passed the night will be appreciated by the day sister, if the night sister has an opportunity of giving it. There should be mutual goodwill and no feeling of antagonism between the two, with a determination on both sides to keep to the duties respectively assigned to them, as far as the nature of their work will permit. Neither dislike of the night sister, nor a special friendliness towards her, should make a day sister needlessly disregard her own time-table, and remain in the wards after 10 P.M. Directly a sister sets aside her own rules, without due cause, she loses ground with her nurses, for it is impossible for her to appeal to them to carry out, from conscientious motives, the regulations laid down, when they see that the same motives do not have sufficient weight to influence her own conduct. But the press of work so frequently occurring during " a heavy take-in " necessitates many exceptions from time to time ; and as, at the London Hospital, the charge of each night sister is too heavy to admit of her taking the day sister's place, for a regular round in attendance on the doctor in any one set of wards, she must not expect the day sister to retire directly the night sister appears, nor attempt to take her place, however much she may desire to help her. If work that should have been finished in the ordinary course of things is

delayed from necessity to a later hour, it means that
the day work has still to be completed, not that it
should change hands in an incomplete condition
because the clock has struck ten. At the same time
anything approaching a regular habit of being late on
duty on the part of a day sister should be sedulously discouraged. It leads to confusion, as day sisters should,
generally speaking, be off duty when night sisters come
on. The hours for day sisters are sufficiently long, and
it is altogether a very undesirable irregularity, except
under the pressure of actual necessity.

The duties attached to the office of night sister in
connection with the domestic arrangements of night
and day nurses and probationers extend the scope
of her power and influence considerably, and afford
valuable experience in general management for any
sister contemplating the charge of a hospital eventually. A great deal of the regularity and general
discipline of the nursing staff in these matters will
depend upon the efficient and conscientious discharge of this portion of the night sisters' duties.
They should be thoroughly imbued with the idea
that it does not rest with them to make exceptions
to any given rule, unless there is a good reason for
so doing, and in that case they must never fail to
report it. Laxity in matters of punctuality and
regular attendance at meals, for instance, creeps
in very rapidly—as all who have had even a brief
experience are well aware—and it is wrong to make
an excellent system futile in practice, by an inefficient
method of carrying it out.

Two years' thorough training does, or should do
more than develop a probationer into a trained
nurse. The regularity of the life, the habit of
working *with* others as well as *for* others, the fact
of regarding oneself, and of being regarded as one
of a number engaged upon the same work, the
importance of doing one's own share well, not only
for one's own sake, but because of the inconvenience
occasioned to others by any failure—all this is a very
important part of the process called "training". It
is not fair that any one of the advantages to be
gained should be lost to those who are not yet in a
position to estimate their value, by any carelessness
of administration. New-comers are apt to think
their own doings of more consequence than the
strict observance of hospital regulations, and to
imagine that an excuse for an irregularity fully
atones for it. The sooner they are undeceived on
this point the better. An excuse is due, of course,
for any failure in duty, but it does not necessarily
justify it, and this is a fact that many probationers
have yet to learn. When they have been taught to
hold themselves responsible for a good result, they
will have made a general principle their own that
may probably render them some service in many
directions besides hospital work.

I do not mean to imply that the sole responsibility
of regulating these matters rests with the night
sisters, for that is far from being the case ; still very
much lies in their hands. The superintendence of
the day nurses' and probationers' breakfasts and

suppers, and of the night nurses' and probationers' dinners, which is required of night sisters, brings them into personal contact with the whole nursing staff. Their supervision should be thorough as well as kindly. It is needless to add that no favouritism should be shown, nor, if it can be prevented, should any opening be given, for the impression that it exists, to be entertained by any right-minded person. Of course, kindness and consideration are due to each one, but unfailing obedience to rule must be scrupulously exacted from all alike. Weak good-nature, and noisy harshness, are equally removed from true kindness, although the former may not appear to be so. A firm, gentle insistence upon the consistent observance of rule, alone renders indulgence possible, when that is desirable, without any fear of such exception detracting from the general discipline maintained.

The failings to which night sisters yield most readily, and against which all new workers in that capacity should therefore be especially on their guard, are—gossip and favouritism—two grave faults that sadly detract from their legitimate influence, and the respect to which night sisters should be universally entitled. They have other temptations, such as failing to report irregularities that they have no right to pass over, lest it might interfere with their personal popularity, but weaknesses of that sort are usually brought to light by other means sooner or later—generally without much delay—and an untrustworthy night sister, being worse than useless, cannot be retained in her office, if the fact of her unworthiness is once known to the authorities. But many night sisters, who are sincerely desirous of performing their duties conscientiously, get into this pernicious habit of gossiping before they are aware. In the course of their rounds they naturally have to listen to a great deal. One sister will do this in a manner to inspire confidence in herself, and to produce a feeling in those who speak, that anything of an unkind or personal nature which they may have said to her, should not be repeated to any one else. Another sister will just as surely encourage gossip by her manner of receiving and repeating it, by her eagerness to ask unnecessary questions, by her manifest desire to " see and hear some new thing," and by her own lack of reticence. As time passes character reveals itself, and each sister will find her discretion appreciated, or her chattering propensities very generally understood, and herself valued accordingly.

Night sisters must refrain from forming gushing friendships with nurses and probationers serving under them, for by so doing they not only tend to spoil the nurse and probationer in question, but inevitably lay themselves open to the charge of favouritism, and thus lessen their influence with those over whom they are placed. If a certain nurse or probationer is known to be " always in sister's room," or sister in her room, at every available moment, it will not only cause discontent, but check any desire others may feel to seek sister's help or advice, on the alternate morning when she is on duty in her own department, and effectually prevent the feeling that she is the friend of *all* her subordinates.

No one will suppose that I wish to discourage genuine friendship, but the manifestations of it must be kept within such reasonable limits as not to interfere with the due claims of a night sister's official influence and position.

I have not intended to imply that these failings are confined to night sisters, but experience has proved that they are more prone to them than the majority of ward sisters. This may be partially explained by the fact that their duties bring them into closer relationship with a larger number of persons, and that all the night nursing staff are off duty at the same hour as the sister, so that in a limited sense there is more leisure for these weaknesses to grow into confirmed habits; but, whatever the cause, earnest workers on their appointment to these responsible posts will do well to be on the alert against such errors as have marred the work of many of their predecessors.

The opportunity which each night sister has for helping those members of the nursing staff who are on night duty is much greater than might at first be supposed. It is true that there are many nights when the sister scarcely has a quiet moment. She seems to be wanted in every direction at once, and has sometimes to make hurried rounds in some wards, in order to give more time and attention to others. But then there are also many nights when the hospital is comparatively quiet, when she can make her regular rounds without finding any urgent or unexpected claims, and when she has time for some little conversation, on matters apart from the immediate needs of the patients, with nearly all who are working under her. She should regard it as a distinct duty to interest herself in the general welfare of nurses and probationers, taking special pains with the progress the latter are or should be making in their hospital studies. That the amount of attention she is able to pay to this portion of her work is necessarily irregular, does not exonerate her from exerting herself in this direction. The *duty* of taking a kindly interest, and of giving judicious advice, is the principle to keep in view and to act upon as opportunities occur.

Without careful guidance a great deal of time will be wasted, either from disinclination on the part of the probationer to exert her mental faculties for her own improvement, or from ignorance of what she had better employ herself with. It is desirable to lose no time in teaching probationers how to apply their energies profitably. There are many instances when a case of special duty affords a great deal of comparatively spare time to the watcher. That a certain amount of this time may be spent in letter-writing, sewing and general reading, cannot reasonably be objected to, but it should not be more than a certain amount. Some nurses and probationers appear to think that as long as they are attending to what may be the very few needs of a patient who still requires watching, that is all that can be expected of them. They forget that they are still "on duty," and should therefore be employing the greater part of such leisure as the nature of their special case permits, for the benefit of the hospital rather than for themselves. If there is no actual work that is required for the hospital under the circumstances, the study of such matters as a good nurse ought to know is a nearer approach to this than occupations of solely personal interest. It is for the sisters, both night and day, to lose no opportunity of representing this to their subordinates; and when all have realised it, time will be more profitably employed, and a definite advance will be made. For the most part night sisters have more leisure than day sisters for answering the many questions which probationers should be encouraged to ask respecting their work. There may be many busy nights together when this statement would seem absurd, but there are also many when the truth of it could be proved over and over again. It is a bad sign when those who are learning have no questions to ask. Both night and day sisters should make their workers feel that this evidence of interest in their work is expected from them. Staff nurses need this encouragement also. They should not be allowed to rest under the delusion that because they have received their certificate, they have learnt all that it is desirable for them to know !

Then night sisters have opportunities of helping the night workers in many respects, besides what may be termed their nursing education. If they will listen patiently to some of the troubles and difficulties, so small in themselves, but so great in their significance to the individuals concerned, they will comfort and encourage them at the same time. I have observed that some sisters grow perplexed as to what line to take when the confidence bestowed upon them implies blame of some other sister. They are sorry for the nurse or probationer, but in their desire to be absolutely loyal to their fellow-sisters, they feel it right to check the confidence which would be given. They act from a right motive, but, I venture to think, not wisely. If sisters remember what a long time it took each of them, individually, to look at the work all round instead of solely from their own point of view, they will not wonder at the struggles that most probationers have to go through before they can do the same. Many a time, if a kind sister allowed a probationer to pour out the tale of her woes, she would find that a sense of injustice was the real source of the trouble, rather than the favour refused, or the remark made, whatever the grievance may be. In the light of a fuller hospital experience it is probable that the sister may be able to represent the matter to the probationer in a manner that, with a limited knowledge of the working of an institution, it was not possible for her to conceive of it before; and, with the apparent injustice explained away, the actual grievance may fortunately be removed. Of course, this may not always be the case, but even if the sister, night or day, be placed in the awkward position of listening to a story in which the sister she would fain uphold is manifestly in the wrong, it would be seldom indeed that she could not think of some kindly excuse to plead on her behalf. At any rate, whilst sympathising with the aggrieved person, she can take the opportunity of impressing upon her the importance to *herself* of bearing the trouble patiently, and of not sacrificing the principle of loyalty, because she may find the difficulty of maintaining it is considerable in her own case. Sisters should have sufficient confidence in their own loyalty to each other, and to the speaker, to enable them to hear what may sound detrimental to another sister, if that becomes necessary, without any fear that what is said to them will do the sister complained of any harm. "Blessed are the peace-makers" is a beautiful saying that should dwell constantly in the minds and hearts of hospital sisters, for there will always be work for them to do in this direction. Before they can make peace they must hear why and how the necessity has arisen, even at the cost of some self-sacrifice. The difficulty of arriving at a right judgment may cause them anxiety, but if their hearts are really full of kindness and charity, they surely need not be afraid of doing any harm with such knowledge as may come to them. It is better for probationers to be able to speak freely to a sensible sister, than to hold forth about their real and imaginary wrongs to companions whose experience is as limited as their own. A sister should be able to trust herself to be silent, unless circumstances arise which make it a duty to speak.

No sister should allow subordinates to criticise other sisters, or to express unfavourable opinions concerning them. In my judgment, there is all the difference between listening to a frank statement of facts, whether they involve blame of a sister or not, and permitting a discussion as to their merits, apart from the case in point. Praise and admiration of a sister's character or work, if it is sincere, need never be checked, for it can hurt nobody, but silence is sufficient for other purposes. A sister should never ask a subordinate how she likes another sister, nor encourage gossip of any description. Still she must forbear to extol what is not admirable, even if it is not necessary for her to say all she thinks in the contrary direction.

A sister who is genuinely anxious to do what is right, and to forward the work to the utmost of her ability, will learn so much from experience in dealing with these matters, that her difficulties and perplexities will gradually diminish, while her power of helpfulness will steadily increase. The path would be frequently smoothed to new-comers if a sister would be a little patient with failings that appear so unreasonable to those who have outlived them. A beginner is perhaps indignant at not being granted some favour that to her appears trifling, and is especially injured at the refusal if consent might have been given without the result interfering with her individual share of the work. An explanation from a sister that in justice to *others* the request was obliged to be denied would probably be a new idea to the probationer. A gentle, but firm reminder that they are not yet in a position to judge of matters, that they are, nevertheless, venturing ignorantly to criticise, would frequently be a help. The fact is obvious, yet many who are willing to accept it, immediately it is placed before them, fail to see it, until it is thus pointed out. It is curious how often we need to be reminded of what we might be supposed to know and remember without assistance.

It is needless to add that before a sister can influence others to much purpose, her example must tend in the same direction as the precepts she gives. There are occasions when her advice may be ignored, but she would perhaps be much encouraged if she could see the definite effect which her example has unconsciously produced.

If a sister endeavours to act towards the authorities of the hospital, with the same loyalty that she teaches to and exacts from her own subordinates, it is manifest that her services will be of inestimable value. In so far as she fails to do this, she herself, and the institution for which she works cannot but suffer. The difficulties of those who are called upon to rule are materially increased if their wishes are met with a disposition to criticise, a determination to oppose suggestions intended for the good of all, or to enlarge upon the obstacles attending their introduction. The mere fact of knowing that *loyal* obedience can be relied upon, and that sisters, who

have so much power to help, are eager to meet the
wishes expressed, will be a great encouragement to
those who are obliged to enforce what is best *for all*,
and who have certainly a right to expect this genuine
assistance from those who serve under them. Cordial
co-operation is such an improvement upon reluctant
obedience. Sisters who are worthy to fill responsible
posts will not fail to realise how much is due from
them.

All those who have to supervise the work of others,
in a greater or less degree, should understand that if
they are not forwarding the work they are distinctly
hindering it. If they do not keep hospital regulations
to the spirit and to the letter, not only will their
own department suffer, but their failures will, in
some measure, detract from the merit of the whole.
If a strict rule, for instance, is made for the guidance
of probationers for their behaviour outside their own
particular wards, the absence of such a rule for the
sisters should not be interpreted to mean that their
conduct need not be characterised by the same
propriety, but rather that their training should have
rendered quietness and decorum habitual to them.
If a probationer sees sisters going about the corridors
noisily laughing and talking together, in a manner
that the former would be severely blamed for, what
effect must it not have upon her? Again, sisters
may see their friends at any time without the order
which alone secures this privilege to their subordinates, because it is assumed that, as head of a
ward, this freedom may be granted to them, without

13

any fear that their work will be neglected, or any
hospital regulations infringed. A rule—and one of
exceptional laxity concerning visitors, as it is at the
London Hospital—necessitates a written order for
the admission of friends of probationers to the wards
in which they may be working. What can we think
of a sister who allows friends to be received without
this order, or even connives at the evasion of a well-
considered regulation, in permitting the friends of
a probationer to obtain admission to the ward by the
subterfuge of asking to see the sister herself? She
slackens the discipline of the institution, and immediately lowers the moral tone of her own wards
by sanctioning a species of deception. By proving
unequal to the duties of her position she shows
herself unworthy of its privileges, and wholly unfitted
for the *trust* reposed in her.

I select these trifling illustrations because a new
sister may be slow to perceive how what she does
inside her own set of wards can affect the general
working of the institution. She may be inclined to
view every exception she is asked to make from the
individual standpoint, and to forget that her department is but a part of the whole. Many other instances
in which the sisters become the practical adminis-
trators of the general regulations of the hospital might
easily be given, but every sister will speedily discover
others in connection with those to which I have
referred.   I have quoted them not so much for their
intrinsic importance as because they serve to show
the manner in which the efficiency of the entire

hospital is influenced, in various degrees, by the competence of each sister.

Another point in which the sister should feel specially bound to set a good example is in paying courteous attention to any visitors to the hospital who may pass through her wards. Whoever may be accompanying them, the sister should at least come forward if free to do so, and see if her services are required, and, in nearly every case, they will be gladly accepted. It frequently happens that visitors may come at inconvenient times, and they are not always pleasant and attractive ; but the fact of their presence in the ward should secure them as much courtesy as a lady would deem it necessary to bestow upon any casual callers, who had a temporary claim upon her time. Sisters will find it necessary to bestow constant instruction upon their subordinates in this respect. A combination of natural shyness, with a failure to recognise the necessity to exert themselves, frequently makes them deficient in courtesy.

It may seem desirable to say something about the consideration which sisters should show to each other, the welcome to a new sister when she needs encouragement, the readiness to render assistance in any emergency, and to give any information which may prevent a mistake, but I believe the existing practice in this respect to be all that could be desired. Except to express my sincere satisfaction that this is the case, and to commend the continuation of these duties to all sisters who may yet join the nursing staff, there is nothing to be said on the subject.

I have spoken much of what is due from the sisters
to every one with whom their work brings them in
contact, but I am also anxious that they shall deal
fairly with themselves. It is more difficult to induce
many of them to do this than might easily be believed.
So little do some sisters care to avail themselves of
the opportunities provided for their recreation, that I
should deem further effort to secure it almost useless,
did I not know that it is an error arising out of the
best intentions, and a misconception of their own
needs.

Some of the most earnest workers are gradually
awaking to the fact that they can do their work infinitely better when they are fresh than when they
are tired, but, as yet, I am afraid some of them are
inclined to ignore this, until they have grown so
overworked that nothing but the hardly-earned holiday prevents a breakdown in health. When they
return refreshed to their wards, they are impressed
with the facility with which they can accomplish an
amount of work that speedily tired them before their
much-needed rest.

It is true that the exigencies of hospital work
necessitate a heavy strain upon the sister's powers
from time to time, but this very fact should teach
her to husband her resources, and not to fritter them
away. All will grow to need their holiday as the
time for it approaches, and the same may be said
of those engaged in every kind of regular work.
But I am very desirous that hospital sisters should
realise the necessity of keeping themselves as fresh

and bright as possible *in* their work, and not only
endeavour to get themselves periodically refreshed to
take it up anew. Even those who have known what
it is to get completely overdone, and are therefore
aware that they cannot tax their powers beyond a
certain extent with impunity, forget that the same
truth applies in various degrees. Nothing but some
recreation daily can supply the energy needed for the
vigorous performance of the daily duties. We may
get through our work very well by making a steady
effort, but we cannot produce the same *quality* of
work even with effort, when we are tired, as we
frequently can do without any conscious effort when
we are in a fit condition for it.

I am confident that when sisters realise more fully
the nature of the various claims which their work
brings upon them, they will find out that they cannot
attempt to fulfil them without taking some steps to
keep themselves from getting depressed and wearied.
If they will once believe that, in spite of themselves,
much of their weariness is reflected upon their work
and their workers, and grasp the fact that the very
work to which they are devoting all their energies,
is suffering by the short-sighted manner in which
they are dealing with themselves, their very unselfishness will induce them to look at the matter
more reasonably.

There is plenty of excuse for never going out, for
a good sister could always find something to do, but
the merit lies in arranging the work so that the
patients find all their wants attended to while the

sister is taking the recreation, that should, if possible, send her back to them refreshed in mind and body. The nature of the recreation is a very individual matter, for it would be impossible to define what constitutes rest and enjoyment to different people. Time off duty should be spent as much as possible out of the hospital, and certainly out of the wards. It is needless to point out that fresh air is a necessity for those who spend nearly all their days in the wards of a hospital. Still the hours of standing which fall to the share of a hospital sister are very fatiguing; and it is easy to understand that resting in her own room, especially if she has an interesting book, or a pleasant companion to change the current of her thoughts, may occasionally be the way of spending her time off duty most congenial to a tired sister. She must avoid the *habit* of using this spare time for finishing up various items of work, though as an exception it may sometimes be necessary.

I would urge upon all those who are engaged, or who are about to be engaged in sister's duties, to take what recreation they can *on principle*, regarding it as a means to an end; the end, of course, being to *maintain* efficiency in their work.

Hospital workers can claim no immunity from the ills common to their fellow-creatures; and if they exempt their lives from healthy conditions, it is obvious that their temper, and their general health will pay the penalty. " I am not tired *of* my work, but I have grown very tired *in* it," was the apt expression of an admirable hospital sister to me once. We should take pains to avert that condition, though, if it exists, we cannot do better than recognise it, and act accordingly. I would have every sister take her allotted times " off duty " as regularly as possible. I would also recommend her to obtain the required permission for taking advantage of such stray hours as opportunity may afford to a good manager. I lay as much stress as possible upon the necessity of taking enough time off duty. I have but little fear of any of our busy workers wishing to take too much, provided they spend such leisure as they can secure in a manner likely to refresh them for their labours. A sister who felt herself at liberty to neglect urgent or special duties for the sake of her own amusement would doubtless be unfitted for her work in many other ways, for selfishness is a very grave defect in any woman holding this post. It is the effort required in arranging to be absent that sometimes deters a sister from going out, when the prospect of so doing is not sufficiently attractive to make the exertion worth while; but this is a weakness to be resisted.

Throughout these pages I have refrained from saying anything about the actual nursiug due from the sisters to their patients, because I am confident that this is a portion of their duties which they are least likely to forget. No definite rule can be laid down as to the amount, or the nature of the practical assistance given by the sister in the carrying out of the doctors' orders; that rests with the sister to decide for herself in every individual case. I would only remind her that this decision *does* rest with herself, and not with her staff nurses, as some appear to think. No slight should be intended, or imagined, because the sister exercises her indisputable right to take any share in the actual nursing that she may deem desirable. How otherwise can she be fully aware of the condition of her patients, and of the manner in which their wants are supplied? I need not insist further upon the importance of exacting a complete report of everything connected with the patients from staff nurses and probationers. Far from allowing this to be a grievance, a clever sister will simply make it a means of actively supervising the comfort of her patients, and of showing appreciation of the manner in which the nurses do their work. But many sisters forget, in their turn, to report all matters of interest connected with their wards, unless they are absolutely obliged to do so. Perhaps they refrain from a mistaken idea that the information is not desired, or that it gives trouble to listen to what is not exactly of vital importance ; but a little reflection would show them that this is an error. A cordial response to the interest felt, and as far as possible shown by the matron in the doings and anxieties of each one, is the best evidence a sister can give that it is appreciated. It is difficult to give and nearly impossible always to afford the support that is constantly needed, if the incidents in question are never mentioned until some complaint has arisen. Besides, it is a duty to supply those with whom great responsibility rests, with such a knowledge of *facts* as may enable them to act to the best of their judgment, leaving as little risk as possible of the unwise decisions that must of necessity occur, if they are arrived at in ignorance of the details of information, which it may be in the power of the sisters to give.

Mutual helpfulness is the desire which should animate all who fill various positions in the same institution, for the achievement of a great work, and as such, the nursing of a large number of patients, with the other duties enumerated, may fairly be characterised. That much *is* steadily accomplished, all who have once been through the wards can testify. Those who have seen below the surface sufficiently to estimate the actual work involved, in producing the results that are apparent, will still more readily acknowledge that there is a great deal to admire.

If I have dwelt chiefly upon what should be done rather than upon what is already admirable, it is not because I am blind to or inclined to slight the merit of what exists, but because so much has now been accomplished, that the attainment of the higher standard, in some respects, which I have ventured to set up becomes a possibility.

It may be an idle vision to contemplate what the work done in our hospital would be like, if the twenty-two or twenty-five sisters of which our total usually consists, were composed of the sort of women I have ventured to depict, as an ideal, but by no means impossible type of a hospital sister. That such a conception cannot be universally realised need scarcely

13 *

detract from the encouragement to be derived from
the fact that, in many cases, it can be confidently
expected, and will be certainly achieved.   Those
who are pleased to indulge in romantic notions as
to nursing the sick may think the practical requirements formidable, but they can scarcely pronounce
the result desired to be less noble than the fancies of
their dreams.   Those who have forgotten their ideal
—if they ever had one—and permitted it to be lost
amidst the prosaic details of their daily work, may
awake with advantage to the fact that a great deal
more than the average fulfilment of routine duties is
looked for from their hands, not only by those who
have no practical knowledge of hospital life, but by
those who can speak of its capabilities, after many
years' experience in it.

It sometimes appears to me as much a necessity for
hospital sisters to free themselves from the prejudices
they have acquired in the early days of their hospital
existence, as for new probationers to disabuse their
minds of the preconceived notions they have formed
as to what it will be like.   " The present is always
greater than the past," and they must recognise the
principle of growth if they would see things clearly
as they are to-day, rather than as they were once, or
as they imagine, or would like them to be.   To look
back upon the past of hospital nursing is to get a
cheering view of what has been achieved, but it is still
more important to find out of what the present and
future are capable.   I have no desire to see our sisters
perfectly contented with things as they are, but in

many respects I rejoice to see them rather turning
their attention to things as they might be. There
are times when I should like to take the liberty of
quoting to a sister the advice of Madame de Lambert
to her daughter : "You must accustom yourself to
think. The powers of the mind are extended and
increased by exercise ; few people make use of it.
How to think is a talent which sleeps with us."

I have studiously endeavoured to avoid any observations which could be construed into reflections
upon the system of training adopted in other hospitals,
and, I shall regret it, if I have made any remarks
calculated to convey an unfavourable or erroneous
impression of our own. I have tried to confine myself
for the most part to setting forth the duties of a
sister at the London Hospital, without wishing to
imply that the methods adapted to that institution
are of necessity best suited to, or even desirable for,
adoption in similar places.

Some suggestions on general management may be
of service in other directions, when others would be
perfectly useless, except to London Hospital sisters,
but I trust these may find hints of a sufficiently
practical nature to repay them for the trouble of
reading what I have written. "Everything in this
world depends on distinctness of idea and firmness
of purpose," says Goethe. That every sister must
possess, at least, some degree of firmness of purpose, is
almost attested by the fact that she has had sufficient
perseverance to gain the experience which, alone, can
give her the technical qualification for the post. I

can only hope that these pages may be of service in helping to form that distinctness of idea which is equally essential to her success.

I cannot wholly conclude without a tribute of heart-felt admiration to some of the earnest women with whom it has been and is my privilege to be associated in hospital work. My convictions of the noble pos-sibilities which this hospital life contains, have been strengthened by the results visible in their personal characters. I owe them the inestimable service of having my best hopes practically realised as to the capabilities of women for doing their *own* work in the world, without injury to their special characteristics. It only remains for others to follow in their steps and

> " Lay up lasting treasure
> Of perfect service rendered, duties done
> In charity, soft speech, and stainless days :
> These riches shall not fade away in life,
> Nor any death dispraise ".

ABERDEEN UNIVERSITY PRESS.